Study Guide for the Generalist Hospice and Palliative Nurse

Editor
Maureen Leahy, BSN, CHPN
Hope Hospice and Palliative Care
Cape Coral, Florida

Assistant Editors
Constance Dahlin, RN, CS, MSN, ANP
Massachusetts General Hospital
Boston, Massachusetts

Judy Lentz, RN, MSN, OCN, NHA
Executive Director
Hospice and Palliative Nurses Association
Pittsburgh, Pennsylvania

HPNA
Hospice and Palliative Nursing Association

KENDALL/HUNT PUBLISHING COMPANY
4050 Westmark Drive Dubuque, Iowa 52004

Development of this Study Guide

has been made possible by the

Hospice and Palliative Nurses Association

ISBN 0-7872-9192-7

Printed in the United States of America

10 9 8 7 6 5 4

CONTENTS

Content Reviewers

Constance Dahlin, RN, CS, MSN, ANP
Advanced Practice Nurse
Palliative Care Service
Massachusetts General Hospital
Boston, Massachusetts

Julie Griffie, RN, MSN, CS, AOCN
Clinical Nurse Specialist Palliative Care
Medical College of Wisconsin
Waukesha, Wisconsin

Donna Hall, RN, MS, M.Ed, CHPN
Director of Education
Hospice of the Comforter
Altamonte Springs, Florida

Michelle Hobbs, RN, MS, CNP
President, Palliative Care Concepts, Inc.
Greenville, Ohio

Douglas Nee, PharmD, MS
Consultant Pharmacist
Pain Management and Palliative Care
Fort Myers, Florida

Carmencita M. Poe, EdD, APN, CS, OCN, CHPN
The Arkansas Hospice
Little Rock, Arkansas

Shirley Ann Smith, RN, MSN, CHPN
Consultant
Dallas, Pennsylvania

INTRODUCTION

In 2001, the Hospice and Palliative Nurses Association turned fifteen years old. This was an important year as HPNA reflected on the changing environment of end of life care. Having moved from hospice care to hospice and palliative care means truly integrating both types of care and state of the art practice promoting optimal practices. In 1994, a practice guide for the hospice exam was developed. This was updated twice.

However, now, HPNA has heard from nurses that they need information, not just for reviewing for the exam, but also to assist them in care. To that end, the education committee examined the Hospice and Palliative Nursing Practice Review and decided it was time to broaden the scope. The result has been to develop a "Core Curriculum for the Generalist Hospice and Palliative Nurse" and a "Study Guide for the Generalist Hospice and Palliative Nurse."

The content of the study guide is divided into three sections. Part one includes practice questions on the broad arena of generalist hospice and palliative care in terms of the physical, spiritual, psychosocial, and emotional care. Part two integrates questions, pain and symptom management within a case study format. Part three focuses on pain management and specifics on types of medications and conversion rates. The result is a wide breadth of topics covered in a manageable format.

The Core Curriculum for the Generalist Hospice and Palliative Nurse and the Study Guide for the Generalist Hospice and Palliative Nurse can be used together to either enter into practice as a novice or to review for the certification examination as a more experienced practitioner. HPNA hopes these resources are helpful to nurses in all settings. We welcome your feedback on whether this meets your needs or if you have other ideas for resource development. We strive to provide useful and pertinent information to promote excellence in hospice and palliative nursing care in all settings.

Constance Dahlin, RN, CS, MSN, ANP
Chair of HPNA Education Committee
Advanced Practice Nurse
Palliative Care Service
Massachusetts General Hospital
Boston, Massachusetts

Editor's Comments

It has been a privilege and a pleasure for me to work with, and be associated with such a fine group of professionals as those who assisted in the development of this study guide. This work represents a magnificent knowledge and passion for the work of Hospice and Palliative Nursing Care. As an outreach of HPNA, what was originally begun as a resource to help nurses prepare for the certification exam, the guide has evolved into a resource for the practice and process of Hospice and Palliative Nursing Care.

Those of us who have been called to the work of caring for the dying are all too familiar with the weight of attention the physical dimension receives during illness in the traditional model of medical care. It has been our great challenge, in hospice and palliative care, to uncover the psychosocial, spiritual, and functional dimensions, however in doing so, reveal the true whole person. This is the true work of caring for the dying.

The information regarding end of life care, symptom management, pain management, and advanced disease is fluid, the progress of our specialty is rapid, and the recognition of the powerfully important work we are doing is becoming self evident. This study guide has been prepared to help the nurse learn and grow, and to help the nurse help others to learn and grow. It is my hope that as your desire to take good care of dying people and their families is enhanced, and as you plug the fundamentals of care into your work, you will see the process of the rewarding and rich profession that is hospice and palliative nursing.

Maureen E. Leahy RN, BSN, CHPN
Clinical Educator
Hope Hospice and Palliative Care
Fort Myers, Florida

Study Questions and Answers

1. In report you are told that Mrs. Jones is actively dying. Her family calls you out at 3 AM because they believe her decline is due to overmedication. As you assess the patient, which findings would most strongly suggest opioid excess?

   A. Decreased level of consciousness and periodic apnea
   B. Myoclonic jerking and impaired corneal reflexes
   C. Miosis and hypoventilation abnormal contraction of the pupils
   D. Periodic apnea and diaphoresis

2. Mr. Hayes is admitted to your hospice program with a diagnosis of AIDS. As you review and prioritize his current medications, you note that gancyclovir should be continued if possible to prevent which condition?

   A. Pneumocystis carinii
   B. CMV retinitis viral infection of the eyes
   C. Toxoplasmosis
   D. Progressive multifocal leukoencephalopathy (PML)

3. Which cancer is the LEAST likely to metastasize to the bone?

   A. Lung
   B. Glioblastoma
   C. Prostate
   D. Breast

4. Which cancer is the LEAST likely to metastasize to the brain?

   A. Breast
   B. Prostate
   C. Lung
   D. Kidney

5. In which disease process are you MOST likely to see spinal cord compression as a disease complication?

   A. AIDS
   B. Colon cancer
   C. Glioblastoma
   D. Lung cancer

1. Answer is B

   A. Incorrect—These symptoms are suggestive of the acute dying phase.

   B. **Correct**—These symptoms are reflective of the toxic effects of normeperidine and morphine metabolites.

   C. Incorrect—Respiratory depression causing hypoventilation may be a significant acute symptom of opioid excess, but rarely occurs chronically.

   D. Incorrect—Periodic apnea reflects neurologic changes with active dying; diaphoresis may occur with temperature change or increased pain, infection or anxiety.

2. Answer is B

   A. Incorrect—Protozoal infections are usually treated with sulfa.

   B. **Correct**—A viral infection attacking the eyes, CMV is most commonly treated with gancyclovir.

   C. Incorrect—Protozoal infections are usually treated with sulfa.

   D. Incorrect—Viral infection causes neurologic deficits currently treated with experimental agents.

3. Answer is B

   A. Incorrect—Lung commonly metastasizes to bone.

   B. **Correct**—Breast, prostate, myeloma, lung, cervix, esophageal, hepatoma, kidney, stomach, testicular, thyroid and uterine cancers are the most common cancers to metastasize to bone. Glioblastoma is least likely to metastastize to bone.

   C. Incorrect—Prostate commonly metastasizes to bone.

   D. Incorrect—Breast commonly metastasizes to bone.

4. Answer is B

   A. Incorrect—Breast cancer commonly metastasizes to brain.

   B. **Correct**—Of this list, prostate is the LEAST likely to metastasize to the brain.

   C. Incorrect—Lung cancer commonly metastasizes to brain.

   D. Incorrect—Kidney cancer can also metastasize to brain.

5. Answer is D

   A. Incorrect—CMV, candida, toxoplasmosis, viral, protozoal, bacterial, fungal infections are most likely to occur with AIDS.

   B. Incorrect—Liver failure is the most common complication of colon cancer.

   C. Incorrect—This is the most common primary brain tumor.

   D. **Correct**—Bone metastasis is common with lung cancer and therefore spinal cord compression can occur at any time.

6. The drug of choice to relieve the patient's feeling of "air hunger" in end-stage pulmonary disease is:

A. Meperidine

B. Lorazepam

C. Percodan

D. Morphine

7. Mrs. Jones has advanced lung cancer and is experiencing new shortness of breath. She has a past medical history of congestive heart failure and has been taking digoxin and furosemide. What is your FIRST action, from the list below, in addressing her shortness of breath?

A. Call the physician to request an order for morphine

B. Hold all medications, position patient in semi/high Fowler's and reassess in 24 hours

C. Inquire if the patient has been taking her medications for CHF

D. Reassure the patient and family that this is part of the normal disease progression

8. Mrs. Smith is 54-years-old and has end-stage ovarian cancer. On your home visit today, she reports a 3-day history of vomiting. She has an increased abdominal girth and reports abdominal discomfort. She also has had no bowel movement in days. Which is most likely to be occurring?

A. Medication side effects

B. Bowel obstruction

C. Spinal Cord Compression

D. Pleural Effusion

9. In reference to question #8, to provide comfort for Mrs. Smith, all of the following choices are appropriate interventions EXCEPT:

A. NG tube to gravity

B. Corticosteroids

C. Metoclopramide (Reglan)

D. Octreotide (sandostatin)

10. Mr. Able is 70-years-old and newly admitted to the hospice program in a long-term care facility. He no longer recognizes his family, is bed bound, and presents with extreme rigidity of all extremities. As you initiate the plan of care, all of the following choices are appropriate interventions EXCEPT:

A. Create an atmosphere with limited stimulation

B. Teach and/or reinforce with facility staff the importance of regular assessments of skin integrity

C. Frequent and gentle stimulation (i.e. touch and music)

D. Encourage family to remain/become involved with care

6. Answer is D

   A. Incorrect—Meperidine should not be used in end stage diseases. Normeperidine is a toxic metabolite of meperidine and should be avoided.
   B. Incorrect—Ativan is indicated for anxiety, which is not the etiology of air hunger in this case.
   C. Incorrect—Percodan would not benefit the neurologic deficit signaling the need to breathe.
   D. **Correct**—Opioids and anxiolytics provide palliative support for symptoms of breathlessness or suffocation. Morphine removes the drive to breathe due to air hunger.

7. Answer is C

   A. Incorrect—This would be unnecessary if it was determined that the patient has been non-compliant.
   B. Incorrect—Holding all medications would not be your first action.
   C. **Correct**—First conduct a complete assessment which includes the patient's reports of compliance with medication schedule.
   D. Incorrect—Since there may be other etiologic reasons, this would not be an appropriate action.

8. Answer is B

   A. Incorrect—Although some medications can cause these symptoms (i.e. vincristine), this is most likely not the cause.
   B. **Correct**—The classic symptoms of bowel obstruction are constipation, distension, abdominal discomfort and vomiting.
   C. Incorrect—Classic symptoms of spinal cord compression are back pain, urinary incontinence and changes in reflexes.
   D. Incorrect—This patient had no respiratory symptoms such as dyspnea, etc.

9. Answer is C

   A. Incorrect—An NG tube would prevent vomiting and therefore provide comfort.
   B. Incorrect—Corticosteroids can relieve obstruction especially if caused by metastatic disease progression.
   C. **Correct**—Reglan® would have no value since this patient has an obstruction.
   D. Incorrect—Octreotide (Sandostatin®) can actually reverse symptoms of small bowel obstruction.

10. Answer is C

   A. Incorrect—This would be an important option. A quiet atmosphere with limited stimulation would be preferred in this situation.
   B. Incorrect—Skin care is a priority in this case due to the extreme rigidity of his extremities.
   C. **Correct**—While music therapy can sometimes be soothing, in this case, frequent stimulation would not be advisable so this could be eliminated in patients with neurologic involvement
   D. Incorrect—We seek to involve the family whenever possible so we would not want to eliminate this choice.

11. Mr. Able becomes less agitated, but claims to see his deceased wife and mother, and hears them asking him to "come home." The family is upset and has asked you to sedate him. What is your response?

    A. Contact the physician and ask for an order for haloperidol
    B. Restrain Mr. Able
    C. Call the chaplain to address the spiritual pain
    D. Assure the family this is normal near-death awareness

12. You are called to the home of a patient with lung cancer who has the following signs and symptoms: headache, facial edema, hoarseness, dyspnea and edematous arms. What is most likely happening with this patient?

    A. Allergic reaction to morphine
    B. Superior vena cava syndrome
    C. Congestive Heart Failure
    D. Pneumonia

13. The process of psychological, social and somatic reactions to a perceived future loss is known as:

    A. mourning
    B. grief
    C. bereavement
    D. anticipatory grief

14. Objective or observational assessment of pain or discomfort in the non-responsive patient includes what indicators?

    A. Behavioral
    B. Psychological
    C. Previous subjective assessment including physical signs and symptoms
    D. All of the above

11. Answer is D

A. Incorrect—There would be no reason to sedate Mr. Able. His family needs reassurance and support as well as education to help them understand what is happening.
B. Incorrect—Restraints would be totally inappropriate and may cause more agitation.
C. Incorrect—While there is a spiritual aspect to this situation, the action of choice is to recognize the normalcy of what is happening.
D. **Correct**—Near-Death Awareness manifests itself in many ways. Mr. Able is approaching death with normal reactions. Near-Death Awareness is associated with dreams or visions of deceased people, God, or heaven; acceptance of immortality may be revealed through talks of a trip or a journey or fear of being alone. One needs to assess the special awareness, needs and communications of the dying, encourage verbalization without judgment or interpretation. One should encourage the family to be present and share important messages with patient, listen for meaning or meaningful experiences, distinguish between "confusion" and symbolic communication (i.e. "going home" may not refer to an unrealistic possibility, it may mean heaven).

12. Answer is B

A. Incorrect—Facial edema, edematous arms and hoarseness are not likely to be related to an allergic reaction to morphine. Allergic responses usually include pruritis and skin flushing.
B. **Correct**—These are classic signs of SVCS, an oncologic emergency requiring immediate attention.
C. Incorrect—Signs of CHF include edema but normally of the lower extremities.
D. Incorrect—Pneumonia does not cause edematous arms and face.

13. Answer is D

A. Incorrect—Mourning is the cultural response to having suffered a loss.
B. Incorrect—Grief is the process of psychological, social and somatic reactions to a perceived loss.
C. Incorrect—Bereavement is the state of having suffered a loss.
D. **Correct**—This is the definition of anticipatory grief.

14. Answer is D

A. Incorrect—Must include all three: behavioral, psychological, and previous subjective assessment.
B. Incorrect—Assessment should include all previous subjective assessments as well as behavioral indicators.
C. Incorrect—Behavioral and psychological indicators should also be considered including signs and symptoms.
D. **Correct**—Behavioral, psychological and all previous subjective assessment information is most helpful in the non-responsive patient to properly assess the current discomforts.

15. Signs and symptoms of imminent death include all of the following EXCEPT:

A. Unable to sleep
B. Declining senses
C. Low blood pressure, weak and irregular pulse
D. Dysphagia

16. The World Health Organization (WHO) analgesic ladder recommends opioids used for severe pain have no ceilings. Acetaminophen, a nonopioid, has a dosage ceiling of _____ per day?

A. 4 Grams
B. 1000 mg
C. 1 Gram
D. 650 mg

17. Which of the following is a non prescriptive management of agitation?

A. Provide stimulating music to divert the person's behavior
B. Speak directly and distinctively into the person's ear to assure they hear you
C. Postpone explanations for events until the person is calm
D. Maintain a calm, familiar environment with minimal stimuli

18. The cultural response to having suffered a loss is:

A. Mourning
B. Grief
C. Anticipatory grief
D. Bereavement

19. When assessing a patient with neuropathic pain, verbal indicators may include the following descriptors:

A. Shooting
B. Aching
C. Dull
D. Localized

84%

80% = 100
85% = 106

15. Answer is A

A. **Correct**—Inability to sleep is not seen in the imminently dying. Quite the opposite is true. The dying person may sleep most of the time due to decreasing cerebral perfusion and metabolic changes.

B. Incorrect—Senses, specifically sight, hearing, touch, smell and taste decline significantly in the imminently dying.

C. Incorrect—Low blood pressure, weak and irregular pulses are seen frequently in the imminently dying due to failing cardiac contractions.

D. Incorrect—Dysphagia appears to be a common symptom in the end-stages of many diseases probably due to muscle weakness and loss of gag and swallowing reflexes.

16. Answer is A

A. **Correct**—This is the maximum daily *recommended* allowance of acetaminophen. One Tylenol® tablet equals 325 mg acetaminophen so twelve tablets would be the maximum allowable dose in a 24-hour period.

B. Incorrect—This equals one-fourth of the maximum daily allowance.

C. Incorrect—This also equals one-fourth of the maximum daily allowance.

D. Incorrect—This equals one-sixth the maximum daily allowance.

17. Answer is D

A. Incorrect—Music should be offered in soft calming tones.

B. Incorrect—Spoken words should be offered in gentle tones to the person.

C. Incorrect—You should explain all events to the person.

D. **Correct**—Maintaining a calm, familiar environment with minimal stimuli is the best non-prescriptive management of agitation.

18. Answer is A

A. **Correct**—This is the definition of mourning.

B. Incorrect—Grief is the process of psychological, social and somatic reactions to a perceived loss.

C. Incorrect—Anticipatory grief is the process of psychological, social and somatic reactions to a perceived future loss.

D. Incorrect—Bereavement is the state of having suffered a loss.

19. Answer is A

A. **Correct**—Shooting pain is the typical descriptor. Others may include sharp, tingling, electrical, burning.

B. Incorrect—Somatic pain is aching, throbbing pain from bone, soft tissue or internal organs.

C. Incorrect—Chronic dull pain is not related to neuropathic pain.

D. Incorrect—Localized describes the location rather than the type of pain.

20. What types of pain typically require adjuvant analgesics?

A. Visceral
B. Somatic
C. Neuropathic
D. A and C

21. What statement made by the patient would cause you to be concerned for possible opioid diversion in the household?

A. "These pills really help my pain—my pain level stays at 2-3 as long as I take my pills like they have been prescribed."
B. "I take four pills each day. Since I have 8 pills left, I need to have my prescription filled tomorrow."
C. "No, I don't have constipation"
D. "My granddaughter is such a big help to me. She makes sure my pills are right there in my pill container ready for me to take at the prescribed time."

22. Mrs. A is a 53-year-old Asian-American who is new to your hospice program. She has a diagnosis of metastatic breast cancer. She reports severe pain (9 on a 10 point scale) in her back and right upper quadrant area. The FIRST thing you should do is

A. Start liquid morphine
B. Start morphine, sustained release
C. Examine the patient and obtain a history
D. Call the doctor

23. When are non-pharmacologic interventions appropriate to use for pain control?

A. In place of opioids, when the patient is fearful of addiction
B. To augment optimal pharmacologic management
C. To keep the family busy so they won't worry about the patient
D. To manage increased pain until the physician is back in the office

24. A 53-year-old man with lung cancer complains of increased pain in his right hip, aggravated by movement and more noticeable at night. When he walks and stands, the pain is greater. He also indicates there is local tenderness on palpation. These are all signs/symptoms of probable:

A. Bone metastasis
B. Impaired bone marrow function
C. Hypercalcemia
D. Paget's Disease

20. Answer is C

A. Incorrect—Visceral pain requires opioids. It is squeezing, cramping pain of internal organs, soft tissues or bone.

B. Incorrect—Somatic pain is aching, throbbing pain experienced in organs, soft tissues or bones and benefits from opioids.

C. **Correct**—Neuropathic pain is generally due to damage to the nervous system. Adjuvants are used to enhance the analgesic efficacy of opioids especially in cases of neuropathic pain. Antidepressants, anticonvulsants, and corticosteroids are examples of adjuvants.

D. Incorrect—As indicated in the explanation for A.

21. Answer is C

A. Incorrect—The patient's pain is well-controlled and she is taking them regularly.

B. Incorrect—Taking four pills per day would mean this person had two more days left in her supply. Filling the prescription should occur soon.

C. **Correct**—Constipation is a normal side effect—having no signs of constipation makes one suspicious for opioid diversion in the household of the person taking opioids.

D. Incorrect—Family guiding drug administration is very helpful and indicates a concerned family member caregiver.

22. Answer is C

A. Incorrect—Liquid morphine is immediate release and can be used for relief of pain but a thorough assessment must be performed first.

B. Incorrect—Sustained release morphine is a long acting agent which requires multiple doses to establish serum steady state. Severe pain must have immediate release morphine.

C. **Correct**—The patient needs to be quickly assessed with a review of her history prior to calling the physician for the appropriate medication order.

D. Incorrect—The assessment must be completed first before calling the physician for appropriate orders.

23. Answer is B

A. Incorrect—The pharmacologic interventions are not replaced by non-pharmacologic interventions.

B. **Correct**—Yes, the non-pharmacologic interventions will augment the optimal pharmacologic management.

C. Incorrect—Pain relief requires pharmacologic interventions; family needs educated to understand pain management.

D. Incorrect—Non-pharmacologics are not adequate for breakthrough pain.

24. Answer is A

A. **Correct**—These are classic signs of bone metastasis.

B. Incorrect—Bone marrow impairment manifests in variations of WBCs, RBCs, and platelets.

C. Incorrect—Hypercalcemia is increased serum levels of calcium and would not cause these symptoms.

D. Incorrect—Paget's Disease is an inflammatory bone disease manifested by bone deterioration. Local tenderness would be an unusual symptom.

25. Respiratory congestion during the dying phase is also known as

A. Death rattle
B. Cheyne-Stokes respirations
C. Apnea
D. Kussmaul's respirations

26. When a patient is comatose, the nurse should

A. Speak to the patient as if he/she were not there
B. Speak to the patient as if he/she can hear
C. Do not speak in the room at all
D. Speak only to family members

27. Agitation should be accurately assessed, because it can be a consequence of

A. Pain
B. Full bladder
C. Fecal impaction
D. All of the above

28. Pathological fracture

A. Always requires hospitalization
B. Must be surgically pinned
C. Can be treated noninvasively
D. Is a sign of poor care

29. Skin that is blistered, cracked or abraded is what stage of skin breakdown?

A. Stage I
B. Stage II
C. Stage III
D. Stage IV

30. What is the appropriate skin care intervention for the skin breakdown described above?

A. Surgical repair
B. Irrigation and debridement
C. Apply protective dressing
D. A & D ointment

25. Answer is A

A. **Correct**—The Death Rattle is caused by respiratory congestion during the dying phase.
B. Incorrect—Cheyne-Stokes is an irregular pattern of breathing commonly associated with the dying process.
C. Incorrect—Apnea is the absence of respirations.
D. Incorrect—Kussmaul's respirations are deep, rapid respiratory pattern seen in coma or diabetic ketoacidosis.

26. Answer is B

A. Incorrect—Dying persons can hear—especially familiar sounds—therefore family and health care workers should be encouraged to continue to speak to the patient in soft soothing tones.
B. **Correct**—One should continue to speak as if the patient hears since it is believed the sense of hearing is the last sense to leave.
C. Incorrect—Patients are comforted by familiar sounds—it is important to continue to speak softly.
D. Incorrect—Patient can still hear.

27. Answer is D

A. Incorrect—All three conditions would cause agitation.
B. Incorrect—Same as a.
C. Incorrect—Same as a.
D. **Correct**—All three conditions would cause agitation.

28. Answer is C

A. Incorrect—Pathologic fractures do not always require hospitalizations.
B. Incorrect—Pathologic fractures do not always need to be surgically pinned.
C. **Correct**—Noninvasive treatment of some pathological fractures would be best in the dying phase, or in patients who are non-ambulatory or poor surgical candidates.
D. Incorrect—Pathologic fractures are a result of the disease process and are not a sign of poor care.

29. Answer is B

A. Incorrect—Stage I is when the skin is deep pink, red or mottled.
B. **Correct**—Stage II is when the skin is blistered, cracked or abraded.
C. Incorrect—Stage III is when there is a crater like wound with involvement of the underlying tissues.
D. Incorrect—Stage IV is when deep ulceration, necrosis, or wet/dry black exudates is present.

30. Answer is C

A. Incorrect—Surgical repair would be used on Stage IV wounds only.
B. Incorrect—Irrigation and debridement is the therapy for Stage III wounds.
C. **Correct**—The therapy for Stage II wounds is to relieve pressure and apply protective dressings.
D. Incorrect—Applying protective dressings is the correct choice. A & D ointment would not be considered appropriate in this case.

31. The state of having suffered a loss is:

A. Mourning
B. Grief
C. Bereavement
D. Anticipatory grief

32. Which of the following is never considered to be a palliative treatment?

A. Blood transfusion
B. Enteral nutrition
C. Surgery to relieve obstruction
D. None of the above

33. Mr. Wilson has dysphagia subsequent to high-dose radiation therapy to the neck area. Which of the following is most appropriate in his treatment plan.

A. Liquids are always better tolerated in these patients
B. Artificial saliva can be used ad lib for dysphagia
C. The side effects of radiation therapy will resolve rapidly
D. For mouth dryness, keep moistened with lemon and glycerin swabs

34. When considering the interdisciplinary approach to symptoms, which of the following is true?

A. Symptom management must first be optimized by team member
B. The team should address all problems at the same time
C. Spiritual pain always presents like physical pain
D. The nurse is the most important member of the interdisciplinary team

35. The most common infection among hospice patients is

A. Pneumonia
B. Septicemia
C. Meningitis
D. Endocarditis

31. Answer is C

A. Incorrect—Mourning is the cultural response to having suffered a loss.
B. Incorrect—Grief is the process of psychological, social and somatic reactions to a perceived loss.
C. **Correct**—This is the definition of bereavement.
D. Incorrect—Anticipatory grief is the process of psychological, social and somatic reactions to a perceived future loss.

32. Answer is D

A. Incorrect—Blood Transfusions could be palliative when the purpose is comfort.
B. Incorrect—Enteral nutrition is definitely palliative in several situations.
C. Incorrect—Surgery to relieve obstruction is palliative to improve the quality of life.
D. **Correct**—All of the above are considered palliative when the intention is for symptom control and not for cure.

33. Answer is B

A. Incorrect—The patient should be permitted to eat whatever he/she can tolerate.
B. **Correct**—Dysphagia is difficulty swallowing. The artificial saliva will make swallowing easier.
C. Incorrect—Side effects resolve slowly.
D. Incorrect—Lemon adds to the mouth dryness and can be painful if there are inflamed areas secondary to radiation. Glycerin has an alcohol base and ultimately worsens dryness.

34. Answer is A

A. **Correct**—The interdisciplinary team must focus on symptom management as a top priority. All other domains respond positively when physical symptoms are alleviated.
B. Incorrect—Problems must be prioritized and coordinated among the team.
C. Incorrect—Spiritual pain may present in any of the domains.
D. Incorrect—All members of the interdisciplinary team are vital. None is more important than the others.

35. Answer is A

A. **Correct**—Pneumonia is common among hospice patients, due to debilitation and decreased mobility, making them high-risk candidates.
B. Incorrect—Although septicemia is a major life-threatening infection, it is not the most common.
C. Incorrect—Meningitis, inflammation of the meninges, would be highly unusual.
D. Incorrect—Endocarditis, inflammation of the endocardium, would be highly unusual.

36. For the patient who has advanced dementia, the priority therapeutic intervention is:

A. Keep TV on to distract patient from wandering
B. Explain every procedure in detail
C. Anticipate safety needs
D. Encourage frequent naps

37. A hospice patient has been on corticosteroids for prolonged periods and exhibits night sweats, weight loss and malaise. He may be exhibiting signs/symptoms of

A. Tuberculosis
B. Hepatitis B
C. Human Immunodeficiency Virus (HIV)
D. Epstein-Barr Syndrome (EBS)

38. A hospice nurse visits Mr. Tuttle, a 70-year-old man with CHF and cancer of the mouth. He is taking multiple drugs, including diuretics, anticholinergics, opioids, tranquilizers, antidepressants and antihistamines. These could cause

A. Xerostomia – dry mouth
B. Stomatitis
C. Dysphagia
D. Esophagitis

39. Mr. Smith is hospitalized with a brain tumor. He is intermittently confused. He has completed a Living Will stating he wishes to have no extraordinary measures. His brother disagrees and requests that "everything possible" be done to prolong Mr. Smith's life. The patient's wishes should be:

A. Ignored because the family member disagrees
B. Respected as written in the living will
C. Discussed with family members and respected
D. Aggressive care should be immediately started

40. The patient lacks decision-making capacity and has no Durable Power of Attorney for Healthcare. He is appropriate for hospice. Which of the following persons could not, under any circumstances, legally sign the consent?

A. A non-related employee of the hospice
B. A next-door neighbor who has known the patient for over 20 years
C. His wife
D. His attorney

36. Answer is C

A. Incorrect—Individuals with advanced dementia should have minimal stimulation.

B. Incorrect—Health care workers should use simple words and explanations with the demented patient.

C. **Correct**—Safety is a major concern and should be a priority with demented patients. Supervision, minimal stimulation and discouraging sleep during daytime hours maximize night safety.

D. Incorrect—One should discourage naps at any time of the day.

37. Answer is A

A. **Correct**—These symptoms are classic for tuberculosis. Immunocompromised patients are at high risk for development of tuberculosis.

B. Incorrect—Hepatitis B is a blood borne disease and is not usually associated with night sweats.

C. Incorrect—HIV is a viral syndrome transmitted via blood from the infected person. HIV in the early stages has few or no symptoms associated with it.

D. Incorrect—Epstein Barr is a virus that is not usually associated with night sweats.

38. Answer is A

A. **Correct**—Xerostomia is dry mouth and can be caused by the interactions of multiple drugs which include antihistamines and anticholinergies.

B. Incorrect—Stomatitis is inflammation of the oral cavity and is not usually caused by these medications.

C. Incorrect—Dysphagia is difficulty swallowing not usually associated as a side effect of these medications.

D. Incorrect—Esophagitis is inflammation of the esophageal lining and is not usually associated with these medications.

39. Answer is C

A. Incorrect—Health care workers have an obligation to honor the patient's wishes as written in the Living Will.

B. Incorrect—The Living Will must be respected but a discussion needs to also occur with the family members to assist and support their concerns while educating about the patient's wishes.

C. **Correct**—Since the Living Will was completed when the patient was competent, it must be respected. Discussing these issues with family members helps the brother recognize these were the wishes of the patient.

D. Incorrect—Aggressive care would be totally inappropriate in this situation.

40. Answer is A

A. **Correct**—The non-related employee is an illegal representative and could not under any circumstance, legally sign the consent.

B. Incorrect—The individual would be legal if the patient named this person as a surrogate decision maker.

C. Incorrect—The wife is the next of kin and therefore is the first to be considered for legal decision-making.

D. Incorrect—The attorney could be a surrogate decision maker if named by the patient.

41. When the patient dies in the home, the Schedule II drugs are

A. Property of the hospice
B. Disposed of by the nurse with a witness present
C. Returned to the hospice or pharmacy for credit
D. Disposed of by any member of the hospice team who attends the death

42. Spiritual care of the hospice patient and family

A. Is provided in accordance with the religion of the hospice chaplain
B. Is only provided by a hospice staff member
C. Is provided to every patient and family admitted to hospice care
D. Identifies and strives to relieve the spiritual suffering of the patient and family

43. Grief refers to

A. The emotional feelings related to the perception of the loss
B. Overt expression of the loss
C. Differences among ethnic groups
D. The state of having endured a loss

44. The extent and duration of grief

A. Are pretty much the same from person to person
B. Vary considerably from person to person
C. Differs considerably between men and women
D. Are the same when death is expected and planned for

45. For grief to be pathological, it must

A. Be more than a year in duration
B. Affect most aspects of the person's life
C. Be preceded by depression
D. Grief cannot be pathological

41. Answer is B

A. Incorrect—These drugs do not belong to the hospice.

B. **Correct**—The drugs should be disposed of by the hospice personnel (preferably the nurse who is responsible for medication management) and witnessed by a second individual as per the written policy.

C. Incorrect—These medications cannot be credited and therefore should not be returned to the pharmacy.

D. Incorrect—These medications should be disposed of by the medical professional responsible for medication management.

42. Answer is D

A. Incorrect—Spiritual care must be provided according to the patient's religion of choice.

B. Incorrect—Spiritual care can be provided by any one known to the patient.

C. Incorrect—Spiritual care is provided according to the wishes of the patient. If they do not wish to have spiritual counseling, it is not required.

D. **Correct**—Spiritual care is intended to relieve the spiritual suffering of the patient and family.

43. Answer is A

A. **Correct**—Grief is the emotional feelings related to the perception of the loss.

B. Incorrect—Grief is an emotional feeling not an overt expression.

C. Incorrect—Although grief differs among ethnic groups, the definition does not reflect ethnic expressions.

D. Incorrect—This definition refers to the mood state of grief which consists of variable levels of sadness.

44. Answer is B

A. Incorrect—Grief is not the same with each individual; many variations exist.

B. **Correct**—Grief has a very individual response.

C. Incorrect—Grief does have gender variability in some individuals but have many other differences as well.

D. Incorrect—The extent and duration of grief has multiple variables.

45. Answer is B

A. Incorrect—One aspect alone does not describe pathologic grief.

B. **Correct**—Pathological grief is complicated and affects all aspects of the individual's life.

C. Incorrect—Depression is just one aspect of grief.

D. Incorrect—Grief can indeed be pathologic.

46. Sarah, a 4-year-old whose mother recently died, is able to play with her friends, laugh and enjoy her toys. Sarah is

A. Obviously depressed
B. Showing disrespect for her mother's memory
C. Grieving normally for a child her age
D. In need of intensive grief counseling

47. In Orthodox Jewish custom, the body is never left alone because

A. Doing so would reflect disrespect
B. Of a lack of trust for health care providers
C. If alone, the spirit may become angered and seek revenge
D. If alone, the family would be afraid

48. The purposes for attending the death of a hospice patient include all of the following EXCEPT:

A. Closure for hospice staff member
B. Confirming the death
C. Provision of comfort and support to the family
D. Prompt removal of medical equipment and supplies

49. Which of the following is NOT a principle of adult learning?

A. Memorization
B. Collaborating
C. Critically reflective thinking
D. Learning for action

50. An example of advocacy in hospice and palliative care is

A. Testifying about the importance of quality terminal care
B. Negotiating continuous care reimbursement with a private insurance company
C. Contacting an airline to get reduced airfare for distant family members
D. All of the above

51. What is the advantage of individual therapy over group therapy?

A. More time for silent reflection
B. Confidentiality
C. Overall, more effective
D. Less costly

46. Answer is C

A. Incorrect—Sometimes intense periods separated by long intervals where they apparently are not affected by the loss.
B. Incorrect—Sarah's behavior is normal and not a sign of disrespect for her mother's memory.
C. **Correct**—Sarah's behavior is normal for her age.
D. Incorrect—Sarah's grasp of concepts related to death, time and permanence are limited and children her age often see death as temporary.

47. Answer is A

A. **Correct**—A relative remains with the dying person out of respect to ensure that the soul doesn't leave the body.
B. Incorrect—This custom does not reflect a lack of trust for health care providers.
C. Incorrect—It is out of respect that the body is not left alone.
D. Incorrect—Answer A is correct.

48. Answer is D

A. Incorrect—This is just one purpose.
B. Incorrect—This is a second purpose.
C. Incorrect—This is an additional purpose.
D. **Correct**—This is not a purpose for attending the death of a hospice patient.

49. Answer is A

A. **Correct**—This is not a principle of adult learning. Principles include collaborating, critically reflective thinking, learning for action, learning in a participative environment, empowering learners, dialoguing in the educational process and self-directed learning.
B. Incorrect—Collaborating is a principle of adult learning.
C. Incorrect—Critically reflective thinking is a principle of adult learning.
D. Incorrect—Learning for action is a principle of adult learning.

50. Answer is D

A. Incorrect—All the choices listed are examples of advocacy.
B. Incorrect—All the choices listed are examples of advocacy.
C. Incorrect—All the choices listed are examples of advocacy.
D. **Correct**—This is the correct answer since all the choices listed are examples of advocacy. Advocacy is considered an important component of professional nursing practice.

51. Answer is B

A. Incorrect—Silent reflection is a partial advantage.
B. **Correct**—Confidentiality is the main advantage of individual therapy.
C. Incorrect—Individual therapy is not necessarily more effective.
D. Incorrect—Confidentiality is the best response.

52. Education is an important part of hospice and palliative nursing practice. Which situations demonstrate education:

A. Publishing in professional journals
B. Attending a national conference
C. Participating in a HPNA chapter
D. All of the above

53. A nurse's role when communicating with a physician is

A. To make him/her see the situation correctly
B. To carry out their orders
C. To advocate for the patient's wishes
D. To suggest an appropriate course of action

54. Appropriate instructions for a 7-year-old hospice or palliative care patient may include statements like:

A. "Drink one glass of water with your pills."
B. "Ask for help when going to the bathroom."
C. "Death is like going to sleep" 7 yr old lack coping skills to c the emotions of death
D. A and B

55. As a case manager, the hospice nurse

A. Supervises the activities of the interdisciplinary team (IDT)
B. Establishes the plan of care
C. Coordinates and oversees the implementation of the IDT plan of care
D. Directs the activities of the other members of the IDT

56. The palliative care patient's primary care physician

A. Turns over the care of the patient to the palliative care service medical director upon admission
B. Usually continues to direct the medical care of the patient
C. Is responsible for overall medical component of the palliative care program
D. Is required to make home visits once the patient is discharged

52. Answer is D

A. Incorrect—All the choices listed demonstrate education.
B. Incorrect—All the choices listed demonstrate education.
C. Incorrect—All the choices listed demonstrate education.
D. **Correct**—All the choices listed demonstrate education, defined as attaining the knowledge to become skillful and competent within a specific body of information.

53. Answer is C

A. Incorrect—Clear communications are vital but the main role is to advocate for the patient's wishes.
B. Incorrect—This is not the main role when communicating—this role would begin following the communication.
C. **Correct**—This is the primary role of the nurse when communicating with the patient's physician.
D. Incorrect—Suggestions are sometimes helpful but the main role of the nurse is patient advocacy.

54. Answer is D

A. Incorrect—This statement is correct however it is not the only correct answer.
B. Incorrect—This statement is correct however it is not the only correct answer.
C. Incorrect—This statement would not be educational for a seven year old patient. Children at this age lack coping skills to deal with the emotions of death.
D. **Correct**—Both statements A and B are appropriate educational statements for a 7-year-old.

55. Answer is C

A. Incorrect—The case manager is not administratively responsible for the team.
B. Incorrect—The plan of care is the responsibility of the entire team not just the case manager.
C. **Correct**—The case manager does in fact coordinate and oversee the implementation of the IDT plan of care.
D. Incorrect—The interdisciplinary team is self-directed. The case manager is an equal member of this team.

56. Answer is B

A. Incorrect—The primary care physician does not turn the care of the patient over to the medical director of the palliative care service.
B. **Correct**—The primary care physician usually continues to direct the medical care of the patient.
C. Incorrect—The primary care physician is not responsible for the overall medical component of the palliative care program—this would be the responsibility of the medical director of the palliative care service.
D. Incorrect—The primary care physician is not required to make home visits.

57. Who must establish the initial hospice plan of care to reflect the Medicare guidelines?

A. The nurse and social worker
B. The IDT and attending physician
C. The admitting nurse
D. The nurse, social worker and the volunteer coordinator

58. Interdisciplinary Collaborative Practice in the hospice setting includes:

A. The coordination of patient care for other health providers
B. Interaction with IDT members at time of admission
C. The understanding that the nurse case manager makes all of the decisions regarding the patient's care
D. The development of the plan of care in collaboration with the patient, family, other health and human service providers and the IDT

59. Supervision of the home health aide or certified nurse assistant includes:

A. Review of the care plan
B. Observation of care being given and teaching an aspect of care
C. Documentation of the supervisory visit
D. All of the above

60. You have been caring for Mr. R for 4 weeks. He was diagnosed with colon cancer 4 years ago and came to hospice for relief of his symptoms of abdominal pain and loss of appetite. You visit once a week. The social worker and chaplain have had phone contact with the wife and daughter, but the patient and family have declined visits beyond the social worker's initial assessment visit. You review Mr. R's plan of care with the patient and his wife at each visit. The following changes have taken place in the past week.

Mr. R is more fatigued, spending more time in bed, and is unable to bathe or feed himself. Mrs. R is also very tired because she is doing more of the physical care of her husband.

What changes would you initiate in the plan of care that would improve quality of life for both patient and family?

A. Provide services of a home health aide if patient/family receptive
B. Counsel his wife on her need to rest
C. Teach his wife how to give a bed bath and make an occupied bed
D. Initiate a referral to the hospice physical therapist

57. Answer is B

A. Incorrect—All team members are responsible for the plan of care.
B. **Correct**—The entire interdisciplinary team and the attending physician are responsible for establishing the hospice plan of care.
C. Incorrect—All team members are responsible for the plan of care.
D. Incorrect—All team members are responsible for the plan of care.

58. Answer is D

A. Incorrect—This choice leaves out the family and patient and assumes coordination *for* rather than *with.*
B. Incorrect—This choice leaves out the patient, family, other health and human service providers.
C. Incorrect—Decision-making is not the responsibility of one individual.
D. **Correct**—Interdisciplinary collaborative practice includes all involved in the case including patient, family, other health or human service providers and the IDT.

59. Answer is D

A. Incorrect—Review of the care plan is just one aspect of supervision.
B. Incorrect—Observation of care being given and teaching an aspect of care is another aspect of supervision along with review of the care plan.
C. Incorrect—Documentation of the supervisory visit is part of the supervision but not exclusively so.
D. **Correct**—All choices listed are part of the supervision of the home health aide or certified nurse assistant.

60. Answer is A

A. **Correct**—This change would be most beneficial for patient and family.
B. Incorrect—Providing assistance will allow the wife to get needed rest.
C. Incorrect—Teaching the wife how to make an occupied bed and how to give a bed bath would not be necessary in this situation.
D. Incorrect—Making a physical therapy referral would not be appropriate in this situation.

61. Knowing that these changes indicate deterioration of the patient's disease, how would you use the IDT to provide coordinated care?

A. Request the social worker and chaplain to call the patient and wife to offer support and to arrange a visit

B. Arrange for equipment and supplies that will make the patient's ongoing care easier for the patient and family

C. Update the plan of care with input from appropriate members of the IDT and the attending physician

D. All of the above

62. Positive steps to help others or to prevent harm is the definition of:

A. Beneficence

B. Veracity

C. Nonmaleficence

D. Justice

63. According to Medicare Hospice regulations, the four members of the core hospice services include:

A. Nursing, physician, medical social services and counseling - dietary, spiritual, bereavement

B. Nursing, home health aid, chaplain, volunteer

C. Whatever is needed to meet the care needs of the patient

D. Physician, patient, family, nurse

64. What dose of morphine can be helpful to relieve cough.

A. 1 mg q 4 hour prn

B. 2-10 mg q 4 hour prn

C. 15 mg q 4 hour prn

D. 12-20 mg q 4 hour prn

65. Mr. Jones is a 58-year-old male with lung cancer. He has good skin integrity but is in bed most of the time. His family has requested a very expensive specialty bed. What ethical principle would you use to determine if the bed should be provided?

A. Confidentiality

B. Autonomy

C. Beneficence

D. Justice

66. The social worker on the team and you do not agree on an approach to a family. Your best response to this conflict would be to?

A. Contact the physician for orders.

B. Become angry and walk away.

C. Go to your supervisor to have him/her resolve the conflict.

D. Work with the social worker directly to resolve the issue

61. Answer is D

A. Incorrect—This choice is just one of the Correct choices.
B. Incorrect—This choice is just one of the Correct choices.
C. Incorrect—This choice is just one of the Correct choices.
D. **Correct**—This is the best choice of those listed.

62. Answer is A

A. **Correct**—This is the definition of beneficence.
B. Incorrect—Veracity is truth telling.
C. Incorrect—Nonmaleficence is avoiding the intentional infliction of harm.
D. Incorrect—Justice is giving others what is due or owed and treating all people fair.

63. Answer is A

A. **Correct**—The core hospice team members providing services are nursing, physician, medical, social services and counseling (dietary, spiritual or bereavement).
B. Incorrect—The volunteer and home health aid are not core members.
C. Incorrect—The core team is specifically those listed in answer A.
D. Incorrect—The patient and family are not the core hospice team although they are certainly the focus of the core team's activity.

64. Answer is B

A. Incorrect—This dose of morphine would be inadequate to control cough.
B. **Correct**—Morphine sulfate 2-10 mg q 4 hour prn would be the appropriate dose.
C. Incorrect—This dose would be higher than necessary to control cough.
D. Incorrect—This dose range would be inappropriate for cough control.

65. Answer is D

A. Incorrect—Confidentiality is the patient right to maintain privacy regarding personal and medical matters.
B. Incorrect—Autonomy is an individual's personal liberty.
C. Incorrect—Beneficence is the duty to help others.
D. **Correct**—Justice is to consider rules and actions that result in fair and equitable use of available resources.

66. Answer is D

A. Incorrect—It would be inappropriate to contact the physician in this situation.
B. Incorrect—Reacting in anger is unprofessional.
C. Incorrect—The issue should be discussed and resolved by the parties involved—the nurse and the social worker. The supervisor should not be involved unless direct resolution efforts fail.
D. **Correct**—Working directly with the social worker would be the best approach.

67. What are the Medicare hospice benefit periods?

A. 30, 90, 90 days
B. 90, 90 and unlimited 90 day periods
C. 90, 90 and unlimited 60-day periods
D. 30, 60, 90 days

68. Which of the following examples would demonstrate crossing of professional boundaries?

A. Making cookies for a patient
B. Going to a patient's birthday party and missing your own son's party
C. Staying an extra half hour to talk to the wife, who is upset
D. Praying with a patient who has requested it

69. Your hospice program is very short on nursing staff and the supervisor has requested you to work on your day off. You are very tired but feel committed to the program. What would be your best response in order to meet the needs of the program and take care of yourself?

A. Suggest the supervisor take care of the patients because you are not going to
B. Let the supervisor know that you are exhausted and need a day off if at all possible
C. Do the extra day without saying anything, because it won't help anyway
D. Throw your hands up in the air and storm out of the room without answering

70. Why is nursing research important to palliative care and to hospice?

A. To meet JCAHO requirements
B. To find a cure for cancer
C. To enhance the art and science of palliative and hospice nursing and to improve end-of-life care
D. To make certain doctors will go along with our plan of care

71. You have been assigned to a new nurse as his preceptor. The most important component of this role is

A. To provide friendship
B. Tell the new nurse how to perform procedures
C. Assist, evaluate and provide guidance
D. Provide networking opportunities

67. Answer is C

A. Incorrect—The correct benefit periods are 90, 90 and unlimited 60 day periods.
B. Incorrect—As stated above.
C. **Correct**—This details the correct benefit periods.
D. Incorrect—The correct benefit periods are detailed in answer C.

68. Answer is B

A. Incorrect—This activity would be within professional boundaries.
B. **Correct**—This example would definitely overstep the professional boundaries of the caregiver.
C. Incorrect—This activity would be well within one's professional boundaries.
D. Incorrect—This activity would be within professional boundaries as long as the patient requested it as indicated.

69. Answer is B

A. Incorrect—This response would be unprofessional and unacceptable.
B. **Correct**—Professionalism requires open communication with your assigned supervisor. Expressing your concerns is important to maintaining open communications and trust.
C. Incorrect—Effective open communications are necessary to maintain trust and effective management. The direct supervisor should appreciate open communication and honesty in his/her workforce.
D. Incorrect—This behavior is unprofessional and unacceptable.

70. Answer is C

A. Incorrect—JCAHO does not require research.
B. Incorrect—Research will help to find a cure for cancer but not all hospice and palliative care patients have a diagnosis of cancer.
C. **Correct**—Research does enhance the art and science of palliative and hospice nursing to improve end-of-life care. It is evidence-based outcomes that assure practice and treatment change if recommendations have a scientific basis.
D. Incorrect—Research is not responsible for making certain doctors will go along with our plan of care.

71. Answer is C

A. Incorrect—Friendship is important to relationship building but it is not the most important component of this role.
B. Incorrect—Precepting should be facilitating and guiding the new nurse not telling them how to perform procedures.
C. **Correct**—Precepting is assisting, evaluating and guiding the new nurse to assure they develop a level of comfort to function independently.
D. Incorrect—Networking occurs whenever new people meet one another but is independent of any precepting responsibilities.

72. Four predictors of imminent death include: not incontinence

A. Death rattle, mandibular movements with respirations, cyanosis of extremities, no radial pulse
B. Mandibular movements with respirations, cyanosis of extremities, no radial pulse, incontinence
C. Death rattle, cyanosis of extremities, incontinence, no radial pulse
D. Death rattle, mandibular movements with respirations, incontinence, cyanosis of extremities

73. Hypoxia manifests itself when the oxygen saturation drops to

A. 95%
B. 90%
C. 85%
D. below 80%

74. The United States opened its first hospice where?

A. Memorial Sloan Kettering Hospice in New York City
B. Hospice of the Western Reserve in Cleveland
C. St. Joseph's Hospice in Boston
D. The Connecticut Hospice in New Haven Florence Wald 1970

75. Which cell type is primarily affected by the AIDS virus:

A. B-lymphocytes
B. Basophils
C. Eosinophils
D. T-lymphocytes

76. What percentage of AIDS patients develop pneumocystis carinii pneumonia?

A. 25%
B. 45%
C. 65%
D. 85%

77. Truth-telling is the definition of:

A. Justice
B. Beneficence
C. Veracity
D. Fidelity

72. Answer is A

A. **Correct**—These are the four predictors of imminent death.

B. Incorrect—Incontinence is not a predictor of imminent death.

C. Incorrect—Incontinence is not a predictor of imminent death.

D. Incorrect—Incontinence is not a predictor of imminent death.

73. Answer is D

A. Incorrect—Must be below 80%.

B. Incorrect—Must be below 80%.

C. Incorrect—Must be below 80%.

D. **Correct**—Hypoxia manifests itself at this level. Symptoms of hypoxia will appear at this level. Patient's family members must be educated to understand the symptoms which may occur at this time.

74. Answer is D

A. Incorrect—Memorial Sloan Kettering is a cancer hospital.

B. Incorrect—Hospice of the Western Reserve opened at a later time.

C. Incorrect—St. Joseph's Hospice is located in London and was the name of the early hospice opened by Dame Cicely Saunders, the founder of the hospice movement.

D. **Correct**—The Connecticut Hospice was founded by Florence Wald (Dean of the Yale Nursing School) in the early 1970s.

75. Answer is D

A. Incorrect—B lymphocytes produce the antigen-specific antibody.

B. Incorrect—Basophils are a type of neutrophil not affected by the AIDS virus.

C. Incorrect—Eosinophils are a type of neutrophil not affected by the AIDS virus.

D. **Correct**—T-lymphocytes have a high affinity for the CD4 cell surface protein.

76. Answer is D

A. Incorrect—Pneumocystis pneumonia is developed by 85% of AIDS patients.

B. Incorrect—Same as a.

C. Incorrect—Same as a.

D. **Correct**—Pneumocystis carinii pneumonia is a very common complication of AIDS.

77. Answer is C

A. Incorrect—Justice is giving others what is due or owed

B. Incorrect—Beneficence is positive steps to help others or to prevent harm.

C. **Correct**—Truth-telling is the definition of veracity.

D. Incorrect—Fidelity is establishing trust.

78. Of the following statements, which is the MOST accurate statement about AIDS dementia?

A. Is caused by the treatment of pneumocystis carinii pneumonia
B. May be completely reversed with antiretroviral treatment
C. Leads to significant cognitive impairment
D. Occurs in all patients with AIDS

79. Fifteen percent (15%) of the AIDS patients will develop which malignancy?

A. Small cell lung
B. Myeloma
C. Lymphoma
D. Kaposi's sarcoma

80. Which of the following statements is TRUE?

A. All cancers are hereditary
B. The etiology of cancer is unknown
C. Cancer is recognized as a two-step process—initiation and promotion.
D. Environmental exposure to carcinogens is always part of the etiology.

81. Which of these cancer modalities has local effects?

A. Chemotherapy
B. Biological modifiers
C. Surgery
D. Radiation implants

82. Which three symptoms describe the early signs of spinal cord compression?

A. Back pain, paraplegia, urinary hesitancy.
B. Back pain, loss of rectal sensation, urinary retention
C. Back pain, leg weakness, "funny feelings" in legs
D. Back pain, decreased level of consciousness, paralysis

78. Answer is C

A. Incorrect—Bactrim does not cause dementia.

B. Incorrect—AIDS dementia is not reversible although retrovirals can delay onset.

C. **Correct**—HIV directly damages the nervous tissue resulting in AIDS dementia.

D. Incorrect—Not all AIDS patients develop AIDS dementia.

79. Answer is D

A. Incorrect—Uncommonly seen in AIDS patients.

B. Incorrect—Uncommonly seen in AIDS patients.

C. Incorrect—Occurs approximately 10% of time—is the second most common type of malignancy seen in AIDS patients.

D. **Correct**—Kaposi's sarcoma is a soft tissue (connective tissue) type malignancy seen most commonly in AIDS patients. It appears as brownish purple circular papular lesions.

80. Answer is C

A. Incorrect—Not all cancers are hereditary.

B. Incorrect—Research continually seeks to define the etiology of specific cancers. Success has been achieved in some cancers. For instance, the etiology of melanomas is the sun.

C. **Correct**—Cancer is recognized as a two-step process. Some initiators include impaired immunologic response, self-repair mechanism is ineffective, viruses irreparably damage cells, and genetic predispositions. Some promoters include family history, smoking, sun, alcohol, diet, radiation exposure, chemical and industrial exposures, etc.

D. Incorrect—Although environmental exposures are responsible for the promotion of several types of cancer, it is not always a part of the etiology.

81. Answer is A

A. Incorrect—Chemotherapy is circulated through the blood stream thereby providing systemic effects.

B. Incorrect—Biological modifiers, like chemotherapy, circulate throughout the body providing systemic effect.

C. Incorrect—Surgery only affects the specific area being treated, although systemic effects in terms of complications can occur.

D. **Correct**—Radiation implants are internally placed and only affect the area where the implants are placed.

82. Answer is C

A. Incorrect—Paraplegia is a late sign of cord compression.

B. Incorrect—Loss of rectal sensation is a late sign of cord compression.

C. **Correct**—These symptoms are classic for early signs of spinal cord compression and require immediate treatment to prevent paraplegia.

D. Incorrect—Paralysis is a late sign of cord compression and the individual's level of consciousness is not affected at any time by the cord compression.

83. Which oncologic emergency is aggressively treated in hospice care?

A. Tumor lysis syndrome
B. Syndrome of inappropriate ADH (SIADH)
C. Hypercalcemia
D. Spinal cord compression

84. The general effects of chemotherapy include bone marrow suppression, alopecia and GI effects because:

A. Chemotherapy is circulated throughout the circulatory system
B. Chemotherapeutic agents affect cells with rapid mitotic rate cell division
C. Bone marrow suppression, alopecia and GI effects occur with all medications of any kind
D. Anti-neoplasic agents kill cells in the bone marrow, hair, stomach and intestines because this is where most cancers originate.

85. Hypercalcemia is commonly seen in late stages of which diseases?

A. Breast cancer, lung cancer, multiple myeloma
B. Pancreatic cancer, prostate cancer, myelomas
C. Colon cancer, glioblastoma, breast cancer
D. Leukemia, non-Hodgkins lymphoma, Hodgkins

86. Breast cancer commonly metastasizes to which sites?

A. Pancreas, bone, brain
B. Lymph nodes, pancreas, liver
C. Lung, liver, bone
D. Brain, bone, spleen

87. A typical patient has smoked how many pack/years before COPD symptoms develop?

A. 1 pack/years
B. 5 pack/years
C. 10 pack/years
D. 20 pack/years

83. Answer is D

A. Incorrect—Tumor Lysis Syndrome is an oncologic emergency secondary to chemotherapy and therefore would be highly unlikely seen in hospice care.

B. Incorrect—SIADH may be treated to relieve symptoms but is not aggressively managed in hospice care.

C. Incorrect—Hypercalcemia may be treated to relieve symptoms but is not aggressively managed in hospice care.

D. **Correct**—Spinal cord compressions can progress to paraplegia if not aggressively managed and therefore even in hospice care is considered an emergency requiring immediate intervention.

84. Answer is B

A. Incorrect—Although this is true, it does not explain why specific cells are affected.

B. **Correct**—Bone marrow, hair and GI cells have rapid turnover due to the rapid mitotic rate and therefore are more specifically affected.

C. Incorrect—This statement is not true.

D. Incorrect—This statement is not true.

85. Answer is A

A. **Correct**—Hypercalcemia is caused by increased bone resorption due to osteoclast activity which is a) stimulated by the tumor, b) a direct result of invasion of the bone by tumor, c) decreased ability of the kidney to clear calcitonin, and/or d) increased calcium absorption from the gut.

B. Incorrect—Pancreatic cancer rarely affects the bones.

C. Incorrect—Glioblastomas rarely affect the bones.

D. Incorrect— Hodgkins rarely affect the bones.

86. Answer is C

A. Incorrect—Breast cancer does not metastasize to pancreas.

B. Incorrect—Breast cancer does not metastasize to pancreas.

C. **Correct**—Lung, liver and bone are the common sites for metastasis of breast cancer.

D. Incorrect—Breast cancer would not usually metastasize to the spleen.

87. Answer is D

A. Incorrect—COPD symptoms occur when the person has smoked more than 20 pack/years.

B. Incorrect—COPD symptoms do not occur this early.

C. Incorrect—Although other symptoms of smoking may occur, COPD will not occur until the person has smoked more than 20 pack/years.

D. **Correct**—The typical patient with COPD has smoked more than 20 pack/years before symptoms develop.

88. Death "rattle" can be decreased by administering:

A. Sympathomimetics
B. Aminoglycosides
C. Anticholinergics
D. Vasodilators

89. Somatic pain is described as:

A. Aching, constant, well-localized
B. Aching, constant, poorly localized
C. Aching, intermittent, well-localized
D. Aching, intermittent, poorly localized

90. What percentage of cancer patients will describe two or more sites of pain?

A. 10%
B. 30%
C. 50%
D. 80%

91. An NSAID is a non-steroidal anti-inflammatory drug. The three beneficial effects from these agents are:

A. Anti-inflammatory, analgesic, serotonin inhibition
B. Anti-inflammatory, analgesic, antipyretic—reduces fever
C. Anti-inflammatory, analgesic, antispasmodic
D. Anti-inflammatory, serotonin inhibition, antipyretic

92. What type of pain would benefit most from amitriptyline?—Elavil

A. Smooth muscle spasms
B. Visceral
C. Neuropathic
D. Somatic

88. Answer is C

A. Incorrect—Sympathomimetics cause vasoconstriction—agents like dobutamine, levophed, neosynephrine, Sudafed®—and therefore would not improve the release of secretions.

B. Incorrect—Aminoglycosides are anti-infective agents and would not improve the release of secretions.

C. **Correct**—Anticholinergic agents inhibit the action of acetylcholine which result in decreased GI motility and gastric acid secretions. The side effects of this group of drugs include urinary retention, dry mouth, blurred vision, tachycardia. These agents should be given at the first sign of moisture because they will not dry up secretions already present. Agents include scopolamine and hyoscyamine.

D. Incorrect—Vasodilators will not improve the release of secretions.

89. Answer is A

A. **Correct**—Somatic pain is aching, constant and well-localized since it causes the activation of nociceptors in cutaneous and deep tissues.

B. Incorrect—Somatic pain is well-localized.

C. Incorrect—Somatic pain is constant.

D. Incorrect—Somatic pain is constant and well-localized.

90. Answer is D

A. Incorrect—The percentage of cancer patients with multiple sites of pain is 80%.

B. Incorrect—same as a.

C. Incorrect—same as a.

D. **Correct**—Cancer patients commonly have two or more sites of pain. Pain relief should be a top priority in symptom management of the cancer patient.

91. Answer is B

A. Incorrect—NSAIDs do not inhibit serotonin.

B. **Correct**—NSAIDs have anti-inflammatory, analgesic and antipyretic benefits.

C. Incorrect—NSAIDs are not antispasmotics.

D. Incorrect—NSAIDs do not inhibit serotonin.

92. Answer is C

A. Incorrect—Amitriptyline (Elavil®) will not benefit muscle spasms.

B. Incorrect—Visceral pain will not be relieved by amitriptyline.

C. **Correct—**Amitriptyline (Elavil®) prevents the reuptake of serotonin and norepinephrine thereby inhibiting the transmission of the pain impulse. Side effects include drowsiness, dry mouth, urinary retention, and orthostatic hypotension.

D. Incorrect—Somatic pain will not be relieved by amitriptyline.

93. Type A COPD is emphysema. The following clinical features are the major symptom of emphysema.

A. Dyspnea
B. Productive cough
C. Normal diffusing capacity
D. Decreased lung capacity

94. "If the gut works, use it" is frequently stated. When pain medications are given via the GI tract, what percentage of patients would get pain relief?

A. 25%
B. 50%
C. 70%
D. 90%

95. Dehydration is very common in the terminal phases of illness. Which of these statements is true about dehydration in the hospice patient?

A. Dehydration is often treated because the patient will be more comfortable.
B. Dehydration is never treated because it has advantages in the dying patient.
C. Dehydration is considered a medical emergency and is always treated.
D. Dehydration is considered a natural part of the dying process and is most often not necessary to treat.

96. Non-prescriptive symptom management for pulmonary disease includes all of the following EXCEPT:

A. Keep room cool and control humidity
B. Move air in room by fan or open window
C. Encourage relaxation by gentle voice, gentle touching and guiding slow deep breaths.
D. Provide oxygen as needed — Rx

97. Complications of water and salt retention are:

A. Hypertension, dyspnea, pulmonary edema, pneumonia
B. Hypotension, dyspnea, pulmonary edema
C. Dyspnea, pulmonary edema, anemia
D. Hypertension, dyspnea, psychotic behavior

93. Answer is A

A. **Correct**—Dyspnea is the major symptom of Type A COPD.
B. Incorrect—Productive cough is the major symptom of Type B COPD.
C. Incorrect—The diffusing capacity is decreased in Type A COPD.
D. Incorrect—The lung capacity is increased in Type A COPD.

94. Answer is D

A. Incorrect—More than 90% of individuals would obtain relief when medications are administered orally.
B. Incorrect—same as a.
C. Incorrect—same as a.
D. **Correct**—If the gut works, use it!! More than 90% of individuals with pain would benefit from oral pain medication.

95. Answer is D

A. Incorrect—Dehydration is truly considered a natural part of the dying process. To treat it would cause more discomfort due to ascites, nausea/vomiting, congestion and the need to urinate more frequently.
B. Incorrect—We cannot arbitrarily state that dehydration is never treated. Patient/family wishes are part of the decision process.
C. Incorrect—Dehydration is not a medical emergency.
D. **Correct**—Dehydration is considered a part of the dying process. Not treating dehydration can decrease cough and congestion, edema and ascites, nausea and vomiting and will decrease the frequency of urination which can actually improve the quality of life.

96. Answer is D

A. Incorrect—Keeping the room cool with control humidity is very helpful and is non prescriptive.
B. Incorrect—Moving the air in the room is very comforting and is non prescriptive.
C. Incorrect—Calm, relaxed atmosphere will assist with symptom management and is non prescriptive.
D. **Correct**—Providing oxygen is a prescriptive method of symptom management since it requires a physicians order.

97. Answer is A

A. **Correct**—These are the four complications of water and salt retention.
B. Incorrect—Water and salt retention cause hypertension not hypotension.
C. Incorrect—Anemia is a complication of impaired coagulation and capillary fragility.
D. Incorrect—Psychotic behavior is a result of metabolic disorders.

98. Advanced symptoms of end stage liver disease include:

A. Fatigue, jaundice, ascites, encephalopathy — early stage of hepatic coma
B. Encephalopathy, elevated albumin levels, fatigue
C. Ascites, fatigue, elevated albumin levels
D. Jaundice, encephalopathy, elevated albumin levels

hallmark symptom

99. Which of the following drugs is not recommended for chronic use because of the risk of accumulation of its toxic metabolite?

A. Morphine
B. Hydromorphone
C. Meperidine — demerol
D. Fentanyl

100. What is the ceiling dose of morphine?

A. There is no ceiling dose of morphine
B. 300 milligrams q 4 hour
C. 600 milligrams q 4 hour
D. 1000 milligrams q 4 hour

101. The state of adaptation in which exposure to a drug induces changes that result in a diminution of one or more of the drug's effects over time is the definition for:

A. Addiction
B. Tolerance
C. Physical dependence
D. Pseudoaddiction

102. When should laxatives be initiated?

A. After the patient has not experienced a bowel movement for five days.
B. When an enema is ineffective.
C. Upon initiation of the opioid.
D. When high fiber, fruits and bulk foods have failed.

98. Answer is A

A. **Correct**—Fatigue is the hallmark symptom of chronic hepatitis. Jaundice appears as the bile builds up in the blood. Ascites is the result of excess fluids, no longer draining through the lymphatics, leaking into the abdominal cavity. Encephalopathy is an early stage of hepatic coma.

B. Incorrect—Albumin levels decrease in end stage liver disease. Liver failure disables the function of protein catabolism.

C. Incorrect—Albumin levels decrease as stated in b.

D. Incorrect—Albumin levels decrease as stated in b.

99. Answer is C

A. Incorrect—Morphine is the "gold standard" for chronic cancer pain.

B. Incorrect—Hydromorphone (Dilaudid®) is very effective with chronic pain.

C. **Correct**—Normeperidine is the toxic metabolite of meperidine (Demerol®). Because normeperidine toxicity often appears after several days of treatment, this drug is not recommended for chronic use.

D. Incorrect—Fentanyl is very effective in specific cases of chronic pain.

100. Answer is A

A. **Correct**—Morphine has no ceiling dose. The dose gradually increases due to tolerance and/or disease progression.

B. Incorrect—Morphine has no ceiling dose.

C. Incorrect—Morphine has no ceiling dose.

D. Incorrect—Morphine has no ceiling dose.

101. Answer is B

A. Incorrect—Addiction is a primary, chronic, neurobiologic disease, with genetic, psychosocial, and environmental factors influencing its development and manifestations.

B. **Correct**—This is the correct definition of tolerance.

C. Incorrect—Physical dependence is a state of adaptation that is manifested by a drug class specific withdrawal syndrome that can be produced by abrupt cessation, rapid dose reduction, decreasing blood level of the drug, and/or administration of an antagonist.

D. Incorrect—Pseudoaddiction is a result of undertreatment of pain causing the individual to appear to be a "drug seeker." In such cases, patients who have suffered prolonged, unrelieved pain may become more aggressive in seeking relief.

102. Answer is C

A. Incorrect—The patient's pattern of bowel movements should be maintained. Opioids decrease intestinal motility.

B. Incorrect—If effective laxative agents are incorporated upon onset of opioid therapy, enemas should not be necessary.

C. **Correct**—Opioids decrease intestinal motility therefore laxatives should be initiated when opioid therapy begins.

D. Incorrect—Although these efforts help with stool evacuation, they are insufficient with opioid administration.

103. In hospice, the patient and family are considered the unit of care. Which statement most accurately describes dying patients and their families?

A. A search for meaning and purpose in life is a common experience for dying patients and their families

B. Dying patients and their families are too consumed with financial problems ever to think about spiritual concerns

C. Dying patients and their families have little to fear because hospice takes care of everything

D. The same care plan can be used for all families because their needs are the same

104. The difference between the origin of hospice and palliative care in the US is:

A. The hospice movement was part of the establishment

B. The hospice movement was part of the city sponsored programs

C. Palliative care grew from academic, teaching hospitals demonstration projects

D. Palliative care movement grew from the community

105. Hospice is:

A. Utilized when nothing more can be done

B. A philosophy of care to improve quality of life for the terminally ill

C. A place where people are sent to die

D. Available to patients and families on weekdays

106. In 2002, palliative care programs are primarily delivered:

A. In the home

B. In the acute care setting

C. In the nursing home

D. In the rehab setting

103. Answer is A

A. **Correct**—Patients and families search for meaning of the individual's life and seek a purpose during the dying phase.

B. Incorrect—Although financial concerns should never be minimized, the focus of the dying patient and their families is not the financial concerns.

C. Incorrect—Hospice provides spiritual guidance to assist the patient and family in finding the meaning of life.

D. Incorrect—Every care plan is individualized therefore no two are alike.

104. Answer is C

A. Incorrect—Hospice was introduced in the 1970s replicating a movement initiated in England.

B. Incorrect—The hospice movement is a national movement not a city-sponsored program.

C. **Correct**—Palliative care units originated in the academic teaching hospitals as demonstration projects. The focus has been to move the philosophy of hospice upstream to encourage the application of the philosophy earlier in the disease trajectory.

D. Incorrect—Palliative care did not grow out of the community.

105. Answer is B

A. Incorrect—Hospice offers symptom management, physical care, emotional care, psychosocial care, spiritual care, bereavement care. Much is done to improve the quality of life for the individual and their family.

B. **Correct**—Hospice is truly the philosophy to improve quality of life for the terminally ill.

C. Incorrect—Hospice is not a building although often there are inpatient hospice units/beds available for respite for acute symptom management. Hospice is a philosophy to improve quality of life for the terminally ill.

D. Incorrect—Hospice is available 24 hours a day, seven days a week.

106. Answer is B

A. Incorrect—Palliative care is currently delivered in acute care settings. Palliative care in the home in the final six months is hospice care.

B. **Correct**—Palliative care is currently delivered primarily in the acute care settings either in a dedicated unit or through palliative care teams.

C. Incorrect—Although nursing homes are perfect for the delivery of palliative care, the movement has not penetrated this setting thus far.

D. Incorrect—Palliative care is inappropriate for rehab settings unless the patient has a life limiting progressively deteriorating disease.

107. The role as of the professional on the IDT is:

A. Well-defined and with specified boundaries
B. Carried out totally independent of other disciplines
C. A reflection of unique expertise that is integrated into a coordinated team approach
D. Performed without personal involvement or emotional attachment

108. Palliative care, provided outside of hospice, can be reimbursed by:

A. Medicare Hospice Benefit
B. Medicare
C. No reimbursement available
D. Limited Reimbursement, including commercial reimbursement, symptoms, ICD-9 codes and other sources.

109. The chaplain or pastoral care person on the IDT is:

A. Always the bereavement coordinator
B. Expected to promote his or her own tenets of faith
C. Expected to be open to a wide range of values and beliefs
D. Responsible for assuring a peaceful death

110. When comparing eligibility for hospice care versus palliative care, the following is true:

A. Both have Federal guidelines for enrollment
B. Palliative care allows for more aggressive therapies
C. Palliative care is not holistic
D. Hospice has a broader enrollment

107. Answer is C

A. Incorrect—The roles of the professionals on the IDT are not well-defined, nor do they have boundaries. Each member of the team is focused on the individual's plan of care and strive to achieve the goals defined by the patient and family. Often this requires crossing boundaries and being very flexible in the role of the team member.

B. Incorrect—The roles of the team must be complimentary to each other not independent of the other disciplines.

C. **Correct**—The team members reflect unique expertise that is integrated into a coordinated team approach focused on the individualized plan of care to achieve the goals as defined by the patient and family.

D. Incorrect—Although team members are charged with the responsibility to function within professional boundaries, emotional attachments do occur and are acceptable within those boundaries.

108. Answer is D

A. Incorrect—Medicare Hospice Benefit does not include palliative care.

B. Incorrect—Medicare does not cover palliative care. There are no DRGs for palliative care at this time.

C. Incorrect—Palliative care has limited reimbursement.

D. **Correct**—Palliative care is reimbursed through the acute DRGs on a limited basis.

109. Answer is C

A. Incorrect—The bereavement coordinator can be the chaplain, a volunteer or any other team member responsible for this care.

B. Incorrect—None of the team members should promote their own tenets of faith. This extends beyond one's professional boundaries.

C. **Correct**—The chaplain or pastoral care person must be flexible and open minded to meet the spiritual needs of the patient and family. Often this responsibility extends beyond the individual beliefs of the pastoral care person.

D. Incorrect—Although the chaplain or pastoral care person is responsible for the spiritual needs of the patient and family, it is the responsibility of the whole IDT to assure a peaceful death.

110. Answer is B

A. Incorrect—Palliative care does not have enrollment guidelines.

B. **Correct**—Palliative care includes whatever therapies are needed and requested by the patient no matter how aggressive.

C. Incorrect—Palliative care is indeed holistic just like hospice care.

D. Incorrect—Hospice care covers the final six months of life—palliative care can cover a much longer period depending on the disease.

111. The side effect of chemotherapy most frequently of concern to patients is:

A. Neurotoxicity—peripheral neuropathies, constipation
B. Nephrotoxicity—blood in urine, renal failure
C. Gastrointestinal symptoms—nausea, vomiting, diarrhea
D. Cardiotoxicity—loss of cardiac muscle tone, congestive heart failure

112. Palliative care is best provided:

A. Alone
B. In collaboration with hospice
C. Only in cancer care
D. Within limited settings

113. Which side effects of chemotherapy can be asymptomatic but has serious life-threatening potential?

A. Bone marrow suppression—especially the white cells, making the patient susceptible to infections
B. Epithelial denudement of the gastrointestinal tract
C. Bone marrow suppression—especially the red cells, making the patient susceptible to anemia
D. Anorexia and weight loss

114. The eligibility for hospice and palliative care is:

A. Six month prognosis for both
B. Six month prognosis for hospice and no time limit for palliative care
C. Not affected by prognosis
D. Not affected by time limits

115. One indication of approaching death is change in the circulatory system, evidenced by the following changes in blood pressure and heart rate:

A. Decreasing blood pressure and increasing heart rate (but weaker) to compensate
B. Decreasing blood pressure and decreasing heart rate (but stronger)
C. Increasing blood pressure and increasing heart rate (but weaker)
D. Increasing blood pressure and decreasing heart rate (but stronger)

111. Answer is C

A. Incorrect—The patient is accepting of neuropathies. Constipation causes some concern but is manageable.
B. Incorrect—The patient does not verbalize concerns for nephrotoxicity. The medical management team seeks to prevent the side effects of nephrotoxicity with intravenous hydration.
C. **Correct**—The patient is most concerned about nausea, vomiting and diarrhea. Nausea is a very distressing symptom and one that the patient fears the most. Stories of old cause anticipatory fears.
D. Incorrect—While cardiotoxicity can be very worrisome, the patient seldom indicates concern for this side effect.

112. Answer is B

A. Incorrect—Palliative care is provided through an interdisciplinary team.
B. **Correct**—Palliative care partners with hospice care to provide the best possible quality of life.
C. Incorrect—Palliative care covers all life limiting progressively deteriorating diseases.
D. Incorrect—Palliative care is best provided through all settings: home care, prisons, acute care, long term care, shelters, outpatient and hospices.

113. Answer is A

A. **Correct**—Neutropenia is silent but dangerous leaving no neutrophils to fight the threat of infections. Neutropenia can be the cause of a septic situation which is life threatening.
B. Incorrect—Denudement of the GI tract is usually very symptomatic with mouth ulcers, heartburn, nausea, diarrhea.
C. Incorrect—Bone marrow suppression is the concern but it is the loss of neutrophils that create the concern with the risk for overwhelming infections not anemia.
D. Incorrect—Anorexia and weight loss are very symptomatic causing great distress in the patient.

114. Answer is B

A. Incorrect—Eligibility for palliative care exceeds six months especially in diseases such as Alzheimers.
B. **Correct**—Although hospice has a six month prognosis, palliative care holds no time limit.
C. Incorrect—Eligibility for hospice care is directly related to prognosis.
D. Incorrect—Eligibility for hospice is directly related to time limit of six months if the disease runs its natural course.

115. Answer is A.

A. **Correct**—As the blood pressure decreases, the heart rate increases in an effort to compensate however due to the approaching death, the heart rate is noticeably weaker.
B. Incorrect—The blood pressure decreases but the heart rate increases.
C. Incorrect—The blood pressure does not increase in approaching death.
D. Incorrect—The blood pressure does not increase in approaching death.

116. To receive palliative care services outside a hospice:

A. Patient must sign consent
B. Patient must sign election document
C. Patient must agree to services
D. Patient has no choice for care

117. Mrs. L is admitted with end-stage cancer, and one of her problems is syncope. Which of the following should be done?

A. Consider discontinuing antihypertensive medications if blood pressure is consistently low
B. Encourage her to remain in bed
C. Encourage her to drink less fluid to avoid needing to go to the bathroom
D. Restrain her in bed so she can't fall

118. Hospice and palliative care

A. Focus on the patient and family as unit of care
B. Focus on the patient as unit of care
C. Focus on symptoms as unit of care
D. Focus on reimbursement

119. It is inappropriate to plan aggressive curative treatment when:

A. Cure is possible
B. There is a realistic chance of worthwhile prolongation of life
C. The side effects of the treatment are more distressing than the potential benefits
D. A patient chooses a clinical trial with informed consent

116. Answer is C

A. Incorrect—The patient need not sign a consent for palliative care.
B. Incorrect—Patients need not sign election documents.
C. **Correct**—The patient must agree to palliative care services.
D. Incorrect—The patient's wishes are the focus of the plan of care.

117. Answer is A

A. **Correct**—Repeated blood pressure readings taken in the lying, sitting, standing positions would provide sufficient information to make a determination whether the anti-hypertensive medications could be decreased or discontinued. With end stage disease, blood pressure naturally decreases eliminating the need for continuing the anti-hypertensive medications. The syncopal responses are usually related to orthostatic hypotension.
B. Incorrect—Although safety is a concern with this patient, we should not encourage her to remain in bed. Education of patient and family should include not ambulating unattended.
C. Incorrect—Fluids are very important to prevent syncopal reactions. Dehydration is a common cause of orthostatic hypotension.
D. Incorrect—Restraining any patient for any reason is inappropriate. Restraints cause a higher percentage of deaths and injury. Avoid restraints unless absolutely a medical necessity.

118. Answer is A

A. **Correct**—The patient and family are indeed the unit of care for both hospice and palliative care.
B. Incorrect—The family is also part of the unit of care.
C. Incorrect—Symptoms are not the unit of care—the patient and family are the unit of care.
D. Incorrect—Reimbursement is not the focus of care in either hospice or palliative care.

119. Answer is C

A. Incorrect—When cure is possible, aggressive curative treatments are appropriate.
B. Incorrect—It is appropriate to plan aggressive curative treatment when there is a realistic chance of worthwhile prolongation of life.
C. **Correct**—It is inappropriate to plan aggressive curative treatment when the side effects of the treatment are more distressing than the potential benefits.
D. Incorrect—It is appropriate to plan aggressive curative treatment when a patient chooses a clinical trial with informed consent.

120. An appropriate criterion for deciding to institute any given therapy for a terminally ill patient is:

A. If the potential benefits outweigh the potential risks or burdens to the patient
B. If the physician wants to try once more for a cure
C. If the family demands it
D. If it will prolong life

121. Palliative nutrition means:

A. Providing whatever the patient desires for comfort
B. Providing sufficient protein, calories, and fat to regain optimal nutrition
C. Providing a low-sodium diet to prevent edema
D. Providing artificial feeding so the patient won't suffer from starvation

122. If the patient decides to revoke the Medicare Hospice Benefit, the patient and family need to know that:

A. Their current certification remains valid if they choose to come back later
B. They will lose the remaining days of the current period
C. They can come back anytime and pick up where they left off
D. Once they leave the program, they cannot come back

123. The dose limiting side effect of morphine in the opioid naive patient is:

A. Respiratory depression
B. Myoclonus chronic muscle spasm
C. Constipation
D. Dehydration

120. Answer is A.

A. **Correct**—If the potential benefits outweigh the potential risk or burden to the patient, therapy should be instituted with permission of the patient.

B. Incorrect—It is inappropriate for the physician to try once more for a cure in the terminally ill patient where cure is not achievable.

C. Incorrect—The patient is the center of decision-making. Decisions to initiate therapies should not be done in response to the demands of the family.

D. Incorrect—The decision to institute therapy should be in accordance to the patient's wishes and according to the plan of care. Prolongation of life is not necessarily providing quality of life which should be the primary goal.

121. Answer is A.

A. **Correct**—The patient receiving palliative care should be permitted to eat whatever he or she desires.

B. Incorrect—Palliative nutrition should not focus on calories or content. The focus should be the patient's wants.

C. Incorrect—Although the education of the patient should include ways to decrease uncomfortable edema, the patient has the final choice in palliative care.

D. Incorrect—Palliative care is providing quality of life according to the wishes of the patient and family. Artificial feeding results in both positive and negative side effects.

122. Answer is B

A. Incorrect—The current certification period does not remain valid if the patient revokes the Medicare Hospice Benefit.

B. **Correct**—The patient will lose the remaining days of the current period if they revoke the Medicare Hospice Benefit.

C. Incorrect—The patient can come back at anytime as long as the criteria are still met, but they do not pick up where they left off.

D. Incorrect—The patient can always come back to the Medicare Hospice Benefit as long as they meet the criteria.

123. Answer is B

A. Incorrect—Respiratory depression is a side effect, however, is not dose limiting.

B. **Correct**—Myoclonus is the chronic spasm of a muscle.

C. Incorrect—Constipation is experienced in all patients receiving opioids, but is very treatable.

D. Incorrect—Dehydration is not a side effect of opioids.

124. Mr. L is a 78-year-old mildly demented male admitted post motor vehicle accident with head trauma and internal bleeding. Mr. L's wife died as a result of the accident. Mr. L has only one living son. Mr. L appears intermittently confused. What should be examined in order to develop a plan of care?

A. Had Mr. L's wife shown signs of caregiver fatigue prior to the accident?

B. His decision-making capacity needs to be determined.

C. Did Mr. L have a living will or advanced directive?

D. What are the son's wishes about Mr. L's care?

125. E. L. is an eleven-year-old Cambodian boy who suffered an anoxic event five years previous to the admission. He has been living in a chronic vegetative state since the injury. Recently he has been developing recurrent pneumonias. The family is now questioning his quality of life. What information about Cambodian culture should the treatment team factor into the care plan?

A. What role does health care take in healing?

B. What is the role of the family in making healthcare decisions?

C. What do Cambodians believe about withdrawing of treatment such as feeding tubes, antibiotics, etc.

D. All of the above

124. Answer is B

A. Incorrect—Decision-making is the main concern to move forward with Mr. L's plan of care.

B. **Correct**—His decision-making capacity needs to be determined. If Mr. L were deemed to be able to make decisions, he would speak for himself. If not, his health care proxy or advanced directive would be used to direct care according to his wishes.

C. Incorrect—Decision-making capacity must be determined first.

D. Incorrect—Although the son is the next of kin, the patients wishes must be honored.

125. Answer is D

A. Incorrect—This is one aspect to factor into the plan.

B. Incorrect—The role of the family is very important, but not the only factor.

C. Incorrect—Withdrawing treatment must be explored with the Cambodian culture along with the other factors.

D. **Correct**—Good palliative care takes into account the role of health and how it is defined in that culture, as well as the family, including how they make decisions and the extent of technology they want used. Some cultures use healers rather that western medicine. In addition, some do not want the body invaded when someone is close to death. The palliative care team needs to elicit this information in order to deliver respectful care.

Case Studies and Answers

Case Studies for Discussion

Case Study #1

Mr. Jones is an 88-year-old man who has been cared for by your hospice for the past month. His admitting diagnosis is prostate cancer with multiple bone metastasis. In the best estimate of his nurse, his rate of physical deterioration indicates that his prognosis is limited to 4 or 5 weeks. Initially, he complained of bone pain in his ribs and pelvis, and rated that pain "4" on a 0-10 scale. Treatment for this pain has been sustained-release morphine, ibuprofen and amitriptyline. Within a few days of initiating this therapy, his pain was self-reported as 0-2, and breakthrough pain was managed successfully with low doses of immediate release morphine. Last week, however, his granddaughter (who works in the health care field) came to visit and talked with him about a new therapy that she has seen "work miracles" on bone pain in men with prostate cancer. Strontium 89 therapy is requested by the patient as a means of pain management. In the nurse's initial discussions with the patient and family about this therapy, she tried to educate them as to the indications and efficacy of this treatment. Complaining about the hospice nurse limiting the patient's autonomy and right to choose, the granddaughter calls the hospice Patient Care Coordinator (PCC) and demands the treatment. As the PCC, you know that this treatment costs around $4,000 to $5,000 total, including hospital stays and other lab costs. This equates to about 8% of the annual operating funds of the hospice. Your hospice is small, with an average daily census of 20 patients and their families.

1. Should the hospice program authorize and pay for the Strontium 89 treatment? Why or why not?

2. Does the hospice have the ability to deny this therapy, even if the patient and attending physician state that it is palliative? Why or why not?

3. Does the patient's wishes supersede those of the hospice? Why or why not?

Case Study #1 Answers

1. **Answer**: As long as the patient rates his pain at an acceptably (for him) low level, and other therapies are effective, the hospice should not pay for the Strontium.

2. **Answer**: The hospice can deny the Strontium treatment; it is a palliative rather than curative treatment, but should only be used if it is the BEST treatment for his pain, or many other treatments have failed. The hospice is obligated to manage the patient's symptoms, including pain, but is not obligated to provide specific treatments, especially when to do so could deplete its finances in such a way that it effects how that hospice cares for the rest of its patients.

3. **Answer**: The patient's wishes are, in the end, paramount. The hospice, however, has responsibility to more than one patient and must weigh how certain interventions impact the bigger picture. The best approach might be for the nurse to help the patient and his granddaughter understand that the Strontium could be considered if all other therapies to control his pain are unsuccessful. It should be clear to the patient and family that his pain and other symptoms will be diligently managed, and that they won't be abandoned by the hospice.

Case Study #2

You are caring for a 79-year-old gentleman with advanced prostate cancer with multiple bone metastasis. He is taking long-acting morphine and at your visits insists he is doing well even though you have noted a gradual decrease in his activity. For example, he used to spend hours in his woodshop; now he rarely goes there. When you point this out to him, he insists he is "fine."

His daughter, however, has a different story. She reports her dad has severe pain and is not taking all of his scheduled or breakthrough medication because, to use his words, "I don't want to die an addict." She has tried to reassure him by telling him it doesn't matter if he's an addict as long as he is getting pain relief.

1. How should you, the nurse, approach this patient and family about his pain and their concerns regarding addiction?

2. What information can you provide both the patient and daughter about addiction?

3. What adjuvant therapy should be considered in this situation?

4. What non-pharmacologic and adjuvant approaches are appropriate to implement in this situation?

Case Study #2 Answers

1. **Answer**: The nurse needs to explore with the patient and family the nature of his pain and how it is impacting his quality of life. She should perform a good pain assessment—duration, intensity, location, precipitating and alleviating factors etc. She can help him see that his pain will change throughout the course of his illness.

2. **Answer**: The patient and his daughter can be helped to understand that addiction is not a danger when a person takes narcotics for the pain of cancer. The nurse can discuss tolerance versus addiction, and also let the patient know that some side effects of the narcotic are transitory.

3. **Answer**: Perhaps the patient would benefit from the addition of an NSAID. Also, one should explore if he can have radiation therapy to any affected areas. Perhaps, also, he is depressed and that has accounted for some of the slowdown in his physical activity; if so, the addition of an anti-depressant might be indicated.

4. **Answer**: The hospice social worker and/or chaplain could visit with the patient to ascertain if spiritual distress or if any unfinished business or fears are components of his physical decline, and offer a volunteer to work in the woodshop for example.

Case Study #3

You are the on-call nurse and are called to the home of a patient who is experiencing the following signs and symptoms: anxiety, sweating, nausea, vomiting, cramps and insomnia. You refer to your on-call information and note the patient is on morphine 5 mg/hour per IV infusion. The patient's wife is concerned that death may be nearing or that her husband is addicted to the morphine.

1. What additional assessment data do you need to gather?

2. What topics may be appropriate to teach the patient and family at this point?

3. What non-pharmacologic approaches are appropriate to implement in this situation?

Case Study #3 Answers

1. **Answer**: These seem to be signs of morphine withdrawal, but the nurse needs to gather data. What other processes could be causing these symptoms (intestinal obstruction? hypercalcemia?). The nurse needs to know the pain history, as well as the history of the morphine infusion. Has the wife altered the rate?

2. **Answer**: It would be helpful for the nurse to probe the wife about her fears; to explain the signs of impending death, and find out if the wife needs additional help. The wife can be helped to understand that addiction is not a valid fear at this point.

3. **Answer**: The wife and patient need to be reassured that they won't be left "alone" in this situation. It might be helpful to have the nurse phone the home every 6 hours or so for a couple of days to see how things are going. If there is reason to suspect that the wife may be withholding morphine, even after counseling and discussion, the hospice might consider continuous care to monitor the situation or an inpatient hospice admission to get the patient stabilized.

Case Study #4

You are called to consult on a new patient who will be discharged home. You are asked to convert her morphine infusion to oral medications. Presently, her pain is well-controlled with morphine 7 mg/hour by SQ infusion.

1. What dose of long-acting morphine would you recommend?

2. What is the appropriate medication for breakthrough pain? What dose would you recommend?

3. What would you recommend for the dose of fentanyl? What medications are most appropriate for breakthrough pain with transdermal fentanyl?

4. What non-pharmacologic approaches are appropriate to implement in this situation?

Case Study #4 Answers

1. **Answer**: 7 mg x 24 hours. = 168 mg morphine IV
   168 mg x 3 = 504 mg oral dose equivalent for 24 hours or 250 mg q 12 hours.

2. **Answer:** Morphine is the correct medication for breakthrough pain. The recommended dose for breakthrough would be 60-75 mg of morphine every 2 hours as needed.

3. **Answer:** Duragesic® 200 mcg with either morphine, hydromorphone, or oxycodone for breakthrough.

4. **Answer**: The patient and family need to be instructed that it takes 48-72 hours for Duragesic® to reach effectiveness and that short-term analgesia (morphine) needs to be taken every four hours until the Duragesic® is effective. Hospice staff should closely monitor patient's pain control and medication side effects in the first critical days after the medication changeover.

Case Study #5

Your new patient is a 30-year-old woman with metastatic breast cancer to the bone and spine. She indicates pain in two places: her right hip and mid-thoracic spine. She describes her hip pain as a deep ache, worse when she walks, and her back pain as a burning sensation that radiates down to her left thigh. Her present medication regimen is acetaminophen and oxycodone (Percocet®) 2 tablets every 3 hours around the clock. Her pain scores (on a 0-10 scale) are:

Pain at its best: hip—4; back—6
Pain at its worst: hip—8; back—9
Pain now: hip—5; back –7

1. What additional pain assessment information is needed?

2. What type(s) of pain do you think Mrs. Jones is experiencing?

3. The physician has asked for your recommendation. How would you change her pain regimen?

4. What non-pharmacological approaches might you try?

Case Study #5 Answers

1. **Answer**: One needs to know how often, in fact, she is taking the Percocet®; how long she has been on this dose; has she had radiation therapy to these areas? Also, what precipitates and alleviates the pain?

2. **Answer**: She is having bone and neuropathic pain.

3. **Answer**: An NSAID and tricyclic, like nortriptyline (Pamelor®) should be started to cover bone and neuropathic pain respectively. Percocet® should be changed to oxycodone 5 mg and dosed at 2 tabs q 3 hour ATC and 1 tab q1h for breakthrough pain. Though this patient was using 16 tablets/24 hours (>4Gm APAP/24h), the addition of adjuvant therapies may decrease the opioid consumption. Consideration of a long acting opioid should be assessed within 24-48 hours after above therapies have been instituted.

4. **Answer**: The patient might benefit from gentle hydrotherapy, as well as planning her ADLs so they are spaced apart and she isn't on her feet for too long at any given time. Perhaps heat and massage might be helpful as well.

Case Study #6

You are caring for a 74-year-old gentleman with end-stage COPD and a history of CO_2 retention. Over the weeks you have known him, he has become increasingly short of breath in spite of countless interventions. You feel low-dose morphine, given as needed, is the next logical intervention. The physician is reluctant to give you the order because of concern over respiratory depression. The patient has never taken opioids before.

1. How might you approach the physician?

2. What starting dose and route would you recommend?

3. How might the patient's family be assured of morphine's safety?

4. What non-pharmacologic interventions are effective for dyspnea?

5. How might the interdisciplinary team be involved with this patient's care?

Case Study #6 Answers

1. **Answer**: You can talk with the physician and explain that morphine's side effects can be lessened by low titration and monitoring by hospice staff. Also, that morphine is especially effective in treating the air hunger of end-stage COPD and that the other interventions have not been effective. Fax research information on use of morphine with shortness of breath to the physician.

2. **Answer**: The recommendation would be to start with 5 mg q 4 hours prn, then titrate up as needed and tolerated. Be sure to ask the physician to write for a stool softener/laxative and an anti-emetic to control the side effects of the opioid.

3. **Answer**: The family should be assured that morphine is used for shortness of breath frequently and that any side effects will be aggressively managed. They should be reassured that the dose will be carefully titrated upwards if necessary, and that addiction is not a concern.

4. **Answer**: The patient might benefit from a fan to circulate air in the room as well as reducing anything in the environment that heightens his sense of being closed in and feeling anxious.

5. **Answer**: The social worker and chaplain may be helpful in talking about the special anxiety that comes with shortness of breath and in helping the patient find ways to be calm.

Case Study #7

You are caring for a 60-year-old gentleman with widespread small cell cancer of the lung, metastatic to the bone and liver. He rates his pain as a "10" on a 1-10 scale, especially in his right hip and leg. You note the patient has a 40-year history of heavy alcohol use (about 10 beers a day, plus some bourbon) and has admitted to some marijuana and cocaine use in the past. He reports, at present, his alcohol intake is less or "a few" beers a day.

1. What additional pain assessment information should be obtained?

2. How would you propose this patient's pain should be managed at this time?

3. If this patient's physician is reluctant to prescribe medications to adequately manage the pain, what resources or help might you turn to?

4. What non-pharmacologic approaches are appropriate to implement in this situation?

Case Study #7 Answers

1. **Answer**: Careful assessment of his pain is needed. When is it worse; when is it better? Is one position better than another? Does he drink to alleviate the pain? What over-the-counter medications has he tried to help with pain? Has he ever been on methadone or any other prescription medication for pain. Has he ever been in a rehab program?

2. **Answer**: The best recommendation is to start by assuring the patient that you are committed to helping him get pain relief. Begin with Ibuprofen 400-600 mg tid and ask him and his caregivers to keep a log of medication administration as well as self-pain rating. If this is ineffective and the physician still won't prescribe anything, ask the hospice medical director to speak to the patient's physician or maybe consider a brief hospitalization or hospice inpatient facility to get his pain stabilized.

3. **Answer**: Radiation therapy, if he hasn't had any; intervention by the social worker to evaluate if there are issues the patient has used alcohol to hide.

4. **Answer**:
   Music therapy consult, chaplain support, directed visualization/relaxation, (Distraction—i.e., funny videos, action movies, etc.).

Case Study #8

You are the case manager for a 62-year-old woman with multiple myeloma with widespread bone involvement. She is presently taking morphine 60 mg every 12 hours. She also has break-thorough medication ordered, and has taken it five or six times per day over the last week. She rates her pain as a "7" on a 0-10 scale. She also has continuing problems with constipation, despite taking a daily dose of milk of magnesia. She is concerned about increasing her morphine dose because of past problems with sleepiness. She reports to you she'd rather be in pain than be drowsy all of the time.

1. What changes would you suggest in this patient's pain management program? Does her breakthrough dose need to be adjusted as well? What dosage would you suggest?

2. Should her bowel program be modified? If so, how?

3. How might you address her concern about sedation?

4. What non-pharmacologic approaches are appropriate to implement in this situation?

Case Study #8 Answers

1. **Answer**: It is important to assess her pain relief with the morphine for breakthrough, and how long, if at all, the pain is relieved. It is also important to assess the type of pain she is complaining of and if it is a new pain. She will likely need the addition of a NSAID for bone pain, and then reassess 24-48 hours after initiation of the NSAID to determine morphine requirements.

2. **Answer**: She needs a stool softener/laxative twice a day, as well as to be reminded to drink enough liquid.

3. **Answer**: It might help her to know that once her body has become accustomed to a higher long-acting morphine dose, she will need less short-acting morphine, and should be less sedated overall. It is important to discuss the addition of the NSAID and it's effect on bone pain, as well as the possibility that she may not need as much morphine to try to control this pain.

4. **Answer**: She needs to be reassured that you will be aggressive and persistent in helping to manage her pain. She might benefit from scheduling activities where pain meds are most effective. Also, perhaps relaxation/visualization sessions would be helpful, or the addition of music therapy. Non-pharmacologic interventions augment the benefits of pharmacolgic intervention but should never be utilized as a substitute for pharmacologic interventions.

Case Study #9

Susan Ryan 2005

You are the case manager for an 85-year-old woman, Agnes, with metastatic breast cancer to the bone, brain and liver. Her present pain regimen is long-acting, oral morphine 120 mg/day with 5 mg MSIR for breakthrough pain. Her primary caregiver is her frail 87-year-old husband, Will. They have lived in a retirement apartment community for several years and have many friends who are already anticipating the loss of Agnes, their dear friend. Agnes and Will are devoted to one another, having been married for nearly 65 years and never have been apart for more than a day. Their three children live out of state but come every month or so to visit and help. Lately, Will is having an increasingly difficult time keeping medications straight and Agnes is often in pain, unable to sleep at night. Several friends who are retired nurses have tried to help, but have warned Will about the "dangerous" medications Agnes is taking. He has called you because he wants Agnes off all of her pain medications, saying, "she was much better before she started with hospice." When you arrive at their home, you observe Will unshaven and overly tired. The apartment is cluttered with laundry, dirty dishes and old newspapers. Both Will and Agnes tearfully tell you they cannot go on much longer. Agnes rates her pain as a "10" on a 0-10 scale.

1. There are many issues/needs in this situation. List them. What is your first priority? Why?

2. Is there additional assessment information you need?

3. How should you, as the hospice nurse, approach them in an effort to achieve better control of Agnes' pain?

4. What might you recommend for Agnes' pain management regimen?

5. What non-pharmacologic approaches are appropriate to implement in this situation?

6. How can the other members of the interdisciplinary team be helpful with Agnes and Will?

7. Consider how hospices define "family." Who are Agnes and Will's "family?" How can (or should) the hospice team support and educate them?

Case Study #9 Answers

1. **Answer**: Issues include uncontrolled pain, exhausted caregiver, "well-meaning" friends, poor understanding of disease progression, patient/husband fear of separation from each other, "inadequate" caregiver. First priority is pain control. Patient and husband will both benefit if the pain is controlled. Then other issues can be dealt with.

2. **Answer**: Can the retirement community offer any extra help in the way of caregiving? Can any of the children come for a time to help? Type of pain, frequency MSIR® used in 24 hours, extent of pain relief if any with MSIR®, and effects of pain on quality of life are additiona questions to investigate.

3. **Answer**: The approach needs to be gentle and both must feel supported. The husband needs to understand that some of his wife's symptoms are due to the progression of her illness and that he can best show his love for her by helping her to be comfortable. He needs to learn the importance of caring for himself, so he can be there for his wife; and to know that those who care about he and his wife can help him with the burden of caregiving. Continuous care, if available, would be helpful for pain management and teaching.

4. **Answer**: This is a situation where either transdermal fentanyl or a subcutaneous infusion of morphine would be indicated. Start with 75 mcg fentanyl or morphine infusion of 3 mg/hour and titrate as necessary. (Would need to assess patient/caregiver comfort with infusion pump.)

5. **Answer**: A hospice social worker as well as all staff can help husband to understand his terror of separation and how important it is that they have quality time together until her death.

6. **Answer**: Volunteer manager and chaplain can be involved to direct friends and family as well as provide respite care.

7. **Answer**: Hospice IDTs usually define "family" as those who are important to the patient. In this case, their friends in the retirement community are as much "family" as any blood relatives. If Will and Agnes wish these friends to help with care, it would be appropriate for them to have some training from the hospice nurse and/or volunteer coordinator.

Case Study #10

You are caring for a patient whose pain has been well-controlled on 45 mg of long-acting oral morphine every 12 hours for the past 3 months. At your last visit, he reports to you increasing pain and the need for more frequent use of his breakthrough medications. He rates his pain (on a 0-10 scale) as 6 (worst), 5 (now) and 4 (least). You notify his physician with this assessment data and request an increase in the dosages of long-acting morphine and breakthrough medications. The physician informs you that he knows this patient well, and all he is doing is seeking medications to escape the reality of his terminal situation. Instead of increasing his oral medications, the physician orders IV morphine to be delivered by an expensive, programmable pump, to ensure control over this patient's opioid consumption. Clinical issues aside, you realize your program's financial officer will challenge the use of this expensive therapy.

1. How might you approach this physician? What other team members or resources can you call upon?

2. What is actually happening to account for this patient's increased pain? Is this addiction? Tolerance? Physical dependence? Opioid pseudoaddiction?

3. What might be important to teach this patient and family?

4. What non-pharmacologic approaches are appropriate to implement in this situation?

Case Study #10 Answers

1. **Answer**: It would be helpful to give the physician specific evidence of the patient's increasing pain and also assure him that hospice team members can address with the patient the reality of his terminal situation. A phone call from your medical director would be helpful. Additionally, if the patient is able to take medication by mouth, that is the preferred route in this situation.

2. **Answer**: In 6 months, his disease has likely progressed. If the patient hasn't exhibited "drug-seeking" behaviors up to now, it seems unlikely he would start. This is a problem of tolerance; he simply needs more medication to achieve the same pain control.

3. **Answer**: To teach the family and patient about how pain changes as disease progresses, but that it can always be controlled.

4. **Answer**: After exploring the specific nature of his pain, the team can suggest the non-pharmacologic approaches that would be most helpful.

Case Study #11

You are performing an initial assessment for admission to the hospice program. Your visit is with a 54-year-old Catholic Filipino man, who has end-stage lung cancer with metastasis to the mediastinum and three ribs. You observe his home to be a small, well-cared-for, yet cluttered house. At the entryway is a Catholic shrine, and inside are many Christian icons. He is oxygen-dependent, and at the time of your visit, he is in moderate distress. After teaching him about a pain scale, he states that his pain (on a 0-10 scale) as 7 (worst), 5 (now) and 3 (least). His current pain regime orders are for acetaminophen/oxycodone tablets 1-2 by mouth every 4-6 hours for pain. He states that he takes one in the morning and one at night. His wife states great concern over his pain, and frustration that he will not take additional medications.

1. Is there additional assessment information you need?

2. What might you recommend for this gentleman's pain management regimen?

3. What role(s) should the other members of the interdisciplinary team play in managing his pain?

4. What patient and family teaching would you incorporate into the pain management plan?

Case Study #11 Answers

1. **Answer**: Find out if this level of pain control is okay with him. Find out if anxiety about his dyspnea is contributing to his distress. Find out what his fears are about. Additionally, is the pain continuous or intermittent, and does one tablet provide pain relief? If so, how much?

2. **Answer**: An opioid such as MS Contin® would be a good regimen since it might also help with dyspnea. Start him on 15 mg q 8-12 hour, with 10 mg MSIR® (morphine elixir) prn for breakthrough. Also a bowel regime and anti-emetic prn orders should be initiated. Since this case doesn't identify the extent of pain and relief: consider the possibility of bone pain and add a NSAID, change Percocet® to Roxanol® 5 mg q 2 hour prn pain and dyspnea. Provide follow up assessment for pain and dyspnea. If the patient is requiring MSIR® frequently throughout the day for relief of symptoms, consider adding MS Contin® to the regimen.

3. **Answer**: The chaplain and the man's own priest might be helpful as the patient is obviously a practicing Catholic.

4. **Answer**: The patient and his family could be taught together the basics of pain control, tolerance, and how pain and dyspnea work together to increase symptoms as well as the use of MSIR® to help both pain and dyspnea.

Case Study #12

You have arrived at JG's house. He has a hospice diagnosis of small cell lung cancer with diffuse metastasis to the bone. He complains of severe shortness of breath, which is NOT cardiac related. His caregiver tells you that lately he has had a tendency to get a little anxious at times. And lately he has become intermittently forgetful and confused. When you arrive you note his vital signs to be BP: 158/88 HR: 124 RR: 26 T:99.

His current medications include:
MS Contin® 60 mg po q 12 hour
Roxanol® 15 mg po q 3 hour prn
Paxil® 10 mg po qd
Albuterol/Atrovent nebs 1 each via nebulizer q 4 hour w/a
Serevent® inhaler 2 puffs bid
Ativan® 0.5 mg 1 po q 6 hour, prn
guaifenisin LA 600 mg po bid

1. What key pieces of information will you include in your assessment?

2. What should be the nurse's first response?

3. What other needs should be addressed?

Case Study #12 Answers

1. **Answer**:
   - Anxiety level? Does Ativan® help? How often does he take Ativan®?
   - Are inhalers used effectively (have the patient demonstrate self administration)? Do the inhalers help shortness of breath?
   - Does the patient have oxygen? What is the liter flow?
   - Does the patient have increased respiratory secretions?
   - Does Roxanol® help with shortness of breath? Is JG using his Roxanol®? How much in 24 hours?
   - Does JG use his medications as prescribed? If not, why not?
   - Do you have a documented pain assessment? Is pain related to anxiety? Shortness of breath?
   - When is the onset, and what is the duration of shortness of breath?
   - What is the lung assessment?
   - Have you done a bowel assessment? Is the patient impacted? Why is there no bowel regime ordered?
   - Mental status?
   - Is the pain exacerbated by shortness of breath? Anxiety?

2. **Answer**: Key pieces of this assessment to manage the presenting symptom of shortness of breath are critical. Anxiety and pain play a role in shortness of breath issues.

   Do a pain assessment to determine how much of the morphine is helpful in the issue of shortness of breath. Look at anxiety as a key component of shortness of breath. Look at breaking the cycle of anxiety/pain/dyspnea in the team approach to care.

   The symptom of shortness of breath, as we are told, is NOT related to Cardiac issues. So the nurse will focus on the primary diagnosis of small cell lung cancer. It is not unusual that this patient has metastatic disease to the bone. There is a high propensity for all lung malignancies to metastasize to the skeleton, and as well, the brain. We understand the implication that bone pain is often unbearable, and must be addressed. Start with an NSAID, a non-steroidal anti-inflammatory drug. This is a missing piece in JG's regime of pain medication. Medications like, Naprosyn®, Indocin®, Trilisate®, Motrin®, Vioxx®, Celebrex® are all examples of NSAIDs. But it is important to have a patient with bone pain on an NSAID.

   Remembering Maslow's Hierarchy one must understand that physical needs must be met first before we move on to psychological, social, and spiritual issues. But clearly having pain and shortness of breath under control is paramount to this person's ability to truly live until he dies.

   Notice his vital signs, notice comfort behaviors, and pain behaviors. Ask the important questions regarding "quality, intensity, duration, frequency." What makes pain better, worse, is it constant/intermittent, what nonpharmacology interventions help?

   JG is taking 60 mg of long acting morphine twice a day (for a total of 120 mg/24). He has taken 8 doses of his Roxanol in the past 24 hours (for a total of 120 mg/24 hours). Therefore his total morphine dose for 24 hours has been 240 mg.

After asking him to rate his pain, "On a scale of 0-10, zero is no pain, and ten is the worst pain that you could imagine, what number would you give your pain?" JG rates it at 4. He states his pain is "0," 20-30 minutes after he takes his breakthrough dose of Roxanol®.

The initial thought might be to increase his long acting dose of morphine, and add a non-steroidal anti-inflammatory drug. Consideration should not be given to the combination short acting opioids. These are the medications that are often a combination of oxycodone and acetominophen (Percocet®, Tylox®), hydrocodone and acetaminophen (Vicodan, Lortab®), codeine and acetaminophen (Tylenol® # 2,3,4), and propoxyphene and acetaminophen (Darvocet-N-100®). It is important to note that these medications have a "ceiling" dose because of the amount of acetaminophen. The recommended dose of acetaminophen must be no more than 4 grams/24 hours, and lower in alcoholic patients, AIDS, patients with liver metastasis, elderly, or those with active liver disease. The third step (ratings of 7-10), calls for the addition of a long acting opioid, such as MS Contin®, Oxycontin®, Duragesic® etc. There is no ceiling dose for opioids so one can titrate to effect.

As a pain-resource nurse we could make a recommendation to increase JG's MS Contin® to 120 mg q 12 hours (as his total in 24 hours was 240 mg and he rated his pain above a 3). An appropriate break-through dose would be 25-50 mg of immediate release morphine (10-20% increase of the 24 hour dose) every 2 hours as needed. As a pain-resource nurse one could recommend the addition of a NSAID and re-evaluate the Roxanol® use over the next 24-48 hours. Then consider increasing the long acting morphine as appropriate.

Once the pain medication dose has achieved an acceptable level of comfort, the next step would be to address the shortness of breath and how it is being treated. One may be able to introduce all his inhalers via nebulizer, and do effective teaching where we are able to document "who we taught, how and when we taught, and indicate understanding by patient or caregiver demonstration. Caution should be given to the total amount of fluid to be nebulized in a given treatment period.

3. **Answer:**

Constipation and impaction are often key factors in the signs evident in JG today. A digital exam is appropriate and necessary. Remember a rule of thumb, that for every 30 mg of morphine, 2 Senokot-S® tablets should be given. Remember that opioids slow transit time. An appropriate daily dose for this patient would be approximately 8 Senokot-S®. If this patient needs a digital exam, do one, with a lubricated, gloved finger, it is done gently and slowly. If the patient is opposed to it, don't force this issue. Rather do a great deal of teaching to make the patient comfortable with this procedure. Use topical lidocaine or certainly premedicate with an opioid. It is a source of dignity and control for many patients.

The choice of stool softeners and laxatives in a patient is important. Osmotic laxatives, should be avoided as they need water "to work." By giving an osmotic laxative (such as lactulose, metamucil, sorbitol) to a dehydrated person the effect of the laxative is reduced. It is better to give a colonic stimulant (senna, bisacodyl, casanthourol) and a fecal softener (docusate sodium).

The other important component of care for this person is the role of the various members of the interdisciplinary team (IDT). Psychosocial, spiritual, functional, and physical needs are made evident in this issue. The disciplines within hospice should address each dimension as it impacts this patient and family. Remember that the unit of care in hospice is the patient and family (whoever the patient defines their family to be).

On to the forgetfulness and confusion issue, remember that cancer cells spread via 3 pathways (blood, lymph and direct contact). Small cell lung cancer spreads rapidly into the blood and lymphatics. It quickly disseminates to bone, lymphatics, brain and liver. If untreated, the average survival time from diagnosis to death is 6 months. The treatment is combined chemotherapy, and it can certainly help prevent the onset of symptoms (pain, cough, dyspnea, hemoptysis, dysphagia, and SVC syndrome), but it is rarely helpful once these symptoms become apparent. Over 30% of these patients will develop cerebral metastasis even after chemotherapy. Understanding this, it is important for you to do a mini mental status exam. The exam has 5 components to it, orientation, registration, attention and calculation, recall, and language. It will allow you to test and score the mental status, giving valuable information to the team. The physician should certainly be notified, and ordinarily the treatment of choice would be decadron (it has an anti-inflammatory effect, and will reduce swelling around lesions in the brain. It will also decrease increased intracranial pressure). Confusion, and headache should improve.

Remember that Ativan® is lorazepam, (in the same family as diazepam, which is Valium®). They both have sedative properties, which is the reason this patient is prescribed Ativan® (for anxiety), but is it the best drug of choice? What about the amnesic effect of Ativan®? Would Xanax® be a better choice for this patient? Ativan® has a relatively short half life, and is excreted quickly, so it is a "cleaner drug" (meaning it has a lower side-effect profile and no metabolites), and may very well be appropriate, but keep in mind if your patient becomes forgetful of historical details, it may in fact be Ativan® at the root cause.

Morphine continues to be the "cadillac" of drugs to treat shortness of breath at end-of-life. The immediate release form (liquid) can be administered by the oral route or nebulized. The long acting form of morphine (MS Contin®) should be considered if a patient requires frequent dosing of the immediate release morphine throughout the day for symptom relief. Oxygen is rarely helpful for patients with obstructive lung diseases, but it will provide comfort. Oxygen is more beneficial in restrictive pulmonary diseases (which JG has).

If one can determine how long JG has been taking paroxetine hydrochloride (Paxil®), and the reason for the medication, it may be helpful to the plan of care. The use of selective serotonin reuptake inhibitors (SSRI) in the management of anxiety related depression and obsessive- compulsive disorder have proven effective. It would be important to refer to the psychosocial professional on your team for follow up and decide whether to increase dose.

Forgetfulness and confusion can be attributed certainly to hypoxemia. Although in considering his primary diagnosis, it would be important to think about hypercalcemia. Lung cancer patients often develop high levels of serum calcium. Hypercalcemia is caused by skeletal destruction (as in bone metastasis), ectopic production of parathyroid hormone, tumor chemical production of prostaglandin, dehydration, immobilization, and hyperparathyroidism. The malignancies most associated with hypercalcemia are: breast, lung, thyroid, kidney, myeloma and lymphoma, and head and neck cancer. A high level of serum calcium is considered greater than 11mEq/L. Symptoms become marked at greater than 16 mEq/L. (Serum calcium levels alone do not always give a true picture. Calcium levels must be adjusted using serum albumin levels to determine corrected serum calcium level. The serum calcium level alone may be misleading.) A serum level of 16 mEq/L is an ominous number, and without aggressive treatment the symptoms are often irreversible. Symptoms that are common are: drowsiness, stupor, coma, nausea, vomiting, polyuria, thirst, dehydration, constipation, fatigue, muscular weakness, diminished deep tendon reflexes, anorexia, paralytic ileus, and seizures. If hypercalcemia were present it would be important to clarify goals of treatment with JG and his family. Treat the underlying cause if appropriate, and treat the symptoms. Early treatments included hydration and diuresis. Presently medications like pamidronate sodium (Aredia®) given IV will bind with free calcium.

One should now look at the complementary therapies and how they may improve the care of this patient. Massage therapy for relaxation and energy work, music therapy for relaxation and refocusing, aromatherapy for relaxation and stress relief, also homeopathic remedies and supplements are often used. When the complements are added to orthodox medical care, the results can be impressive. They must be used appropriately with attention to cultural considerations.

4. Non-pharmacologic interventions include, perhaps, a small fan placed in front of JG, as cool air blowing at him may give him a sense of breathfulness. In warm climates, place a bowl of ice in front of the fan and you can make a little air conditioner!

Case Study #13

KC is a 36-year-old woman with a diagnosis of colon cancer with multiple sites of metastatic disease to the liver, and lymph nodes. When you arrive at her home her husband and 2 children are present. You learn that she has been lethargic and confused at times. She has had surgery, and chemotherapy (last treatment 3 months ago). On your assessment you identify:

- recent mild nausea
- poor appetite
- no BM for 4 days
- c/o lower back pain Visual Analog Scale = 6/10 not relieved by Tylox®, of which she takes 2 caps every 3 hours around the clock
- functional status Karnofsky score of 50
- the rectal vault is empty, and she has rare, sluggish bowel sounds.
- you note evidence of ascites, hepatomegaly, and a tender lower abdomen
- she is jaundiced, and her skin is cool and clammy
- she appears frightened, confused, and clumsy. She is not able to perform the elements of the mini mental status exam
- BP 110/54 HR 104 RR 24 T 99
- Her current medications include:
    - psyllium (Metamucil®)
    - metoclopramide hydrochloride (Reglan®)
    - lorazepam (Ativan®)
    - fluoxetine hydrochloride (Prozac®)
    - megestrol acetate (Megace®)
    - oxycodone 5 mg/APAP 500 mg (Tylox®)
    - Maalox

1. What is the main issue in this situation?

2. What interventions/actions would you take? What recommendations would you make? What should be the nurse's first response?

3. What other needs should be addressed?

Case Study #13 Answers

1. **Answer:**
   There are many issues present in this case. First look at the profile of metastatic colon cancer. The classic presentation of colon cancer is altered bowel habits with the presence of mucous or blood in the stool. There is often not a palpable mass in the abdomen. Tumors generally found on the right side on the colon (ascending) rarely obstruct and usually present with anemia and weight loss. Tumors arising in the left colon (descending) often are obstructive, bulky, present with colicky pain and often perforate the bowel wall. A unique thing about colon cancer is that it spreads directly into the surrounding structures such as the mesentery, and retroperitoneal cavity. The spread to the liver occurs via the bloodstream (the colon sits directly on top of the hepatic artery). The issues of pain, intestinal obstruction, ascites, and high ammonia levels are common in advanced disease states, where hepatic metastasis is present.

2. **Answer:**
   Confusion and Lethargy:
   High ammonia levels are common in liver disease, more often associated with cirrhosis of the liver, but can be seen in metastatic disease to the liver such as in KC's case. Lactulose is the drug of choice as it is metabolized by gut bacteria to acetic and lactic acids which prevent bacterial conversion of urea to ammonia. Lactulose causes diarrhea, thus reducing ammonia levels. Cardinal signs of increased ammonia levels are confusion, profound lethargy, alterations in consciousness levels, jaundice is usually present, tremors, as well as cool and clammy skin. High ammonia levels can be a terminal event, without treatment. Sleep and obtundation come quickly. Treatment may be appropriate in this case.

   Pain:
   It is most important to look at the whole picture of KC's situation. Are there signs and symptoms pointing toward end of life? The IDT must be looking at things like early bereavement for the children, personal affairs and advance care planning completed, spiritual and psychosocial care in place.

   KC has rated her pain at 6 on the numeric intensity scale. Her daily dose of Tylox® has been 2 tablets every 3 hours around-the-clock (ATC).

   1 Tylox® = 5 mg of oxycodone + 500 mg of acetaminophen. Her total daily intake equals (2 tabs x 8 doses). We see that she has taken 80mg of oxycodone + 8000 mg of acetaminophen! This dose is 4000 mg over the recommended ceiling dose of acetaminophen! In the presence of liver disease this is a critical dose. Therefore, we should convert her oxycodone/APAP to a single opioid agent.

   For example purposes, we will convert to oral morphine:

   We know that 30mg of oral morphine is equivalent to 20mg of oral oxycodone bid so our formula should look like this:

   30 mg morphine: x mg morphine/24 hours

   20 mg oxycodone: 80 mg oxycodone/24 hours

   $20x = 2400$

   $x = 120$ mg morphine/24 hours.

KC's equivalent morphine dose in 24 hours is 120 mg; divided into a 12-hour dose (as MS Contin® pain and adjust for her pain at level 6/10 by increasing the q 12 hour dose by 25-50%, her dose would be 75 mg of MS Contin® q 12 hour.

Since she rates her pain at "6," it would be critical to give her breakthrough doses.

The appropriate breakthrough dose is 10-20% of the 24-hour dose, therefore her dose would be 15–30 mg of MSIR q 2 hour prn

Her morphine order should look like this:

75 mg MS Contin® q 12 hour with 15–30 mg MSIR q 2 hour prn for breakthrough pain.

Good pain management is about assessment and re-assessment. The use of non-pharmacologic interventions should never preclude appropriate use of medications, including opioids. Some things to think about are:

- encouraging the patient to remain active and participate in self-care, cutaneous stimulation to reduce muscle tension or spasm, psychosocial and pastoral care,
- heat/cold,
- relaxation and imagery to include meditation,
- music therapy,
- aromatherapy,
- acupuncture,
- massage,
- energy work,
- distraction and re-framing techniques,
- high levels of education for the patient and family regarding pain issues,
- management and goals of treatment,
- peer support groups,
- setting realistic goals re: expectations and outcomes and adjuvants like radiation therapy, strontium 89, ablative surgeries, nerve blocks, etc.

It is important to never forget to include in our assessment the effect pain has on quality of life, and what the effects of pain are on mood, sleep, movement, and appetite. After symptom management is addressed, advanced directives and DNR status need to be discussed.

Bowels:
Assessment reveals no BM for 4 days, poor appetite, and nausea. KC is taking Metamucil®, Maalox®, Reglan®, and Megace®. Her skin is cool and clammy. She is hypotensive with an increased heart rate; rectal vault is empty and ballooned, with rare sluggish bowel sounds. Ascites and distention are present, and she has low back pain, and abdominal tenderness on palpation. She has not eaten in days. This may be a picture of bowel obstruction.

Bowel obstruction occurs most commonly in ovarian and colon cancers. Occasionally it may occur in malignancies such as endometrial, prostate, lymphomas, bladder and stomach. Symptoms can include: continuous pain, nausea, vomiting, constipation, diarrhea, colicky pain, anorexia, and confusion. An empty ballooned rectum on rectal exam can be a sign of impaction with feces higher up in the colon. Remembering that severe constipation can mimic obstruction, the exam is important. The treatment for constipation is a stool softener and a stimulant (i.e., Senokot-S®). Dulcolox and an enema are appropriate here, with a timely reassessment of results. Metamucil is a poor choice for KC as it may add bulk to her stool, and prevent evacuation from a lack of fluids intake. Her bowel regime has been weak, as she has been taking opioids for pain. The rule of thumb is that patients on opioids should begin a bowel regimen with a softener and a bowel stimulant.

A patient should have a BM every three days regardless of intake. Another rule of thumb is for every 30mg of opioid the person should be on 2 Senokot-S® tabs. There is no "ceiling" dose for Senokot-S®, but the patient may not tolerate so many pills! In this case consider adding lactulose, MOM, glycerine, or switching regimens to Dulcolax® or Miralax®.

The last issue regarding bowels has to do with Reglan® (metoclopromide). Remembering that Reglan® causes an increase in motility of the upper GI tract, in the case of possible obstruction KC should be taken off her metoclopromide. A side effect of metoclopromide can be diarrhea, and so it may be of benefit in the absence of obstruction. It is important to know the etiology of nausea. Is the vomiting center being affected via the CTZ? Vestibular apparatus? Cerebral Cortex? or vagal stimulus? Each type of nausea requires a different approach. Compazine®, Decadron®, as well as Reglan® (in the ABSENCE of obstruction) all are appropriate choices. If your agency uses combination suppositories and transdermal gels they may be even more helpful than single agents.

3. **Answer:**
When Megace® was first used to treat post-menopausal women with breast cancer as a synthetic progestin with antineoplastic properties, it caused weight gain and appetite stimulation. Hence it is use as an appetite stimulant for patients with anorexia and cachexia. Ordinarily if Megace® is not helpful after a 2-week trial (maximum daily dose of 800 mg) as an appetite stimulant, it is appropriate to stop. Other choices are Ritalin® to increase mood and appetite. In the case of KC we may want to discuss the issues of eating with the team, and encourage this family to "make it ok not to eat." It is rare that KC would have an appetite at all, if allowed to express her true feelings.

Case Study #14

Mr. L is a 54-year-old man with ALS. He was diagnosed 6 years ago and has been receiving care at home. He is bedridden at home on BIPAP and receives frequent suctioning. He has devoted caregivers and his skin is intact without any bedsores. When he begins to have more periods of distress, his caregivers suggest a palliative care team. Hospice is suggested, however, none in the area support having the patient on a ventilator, as they see that as life-sustaining therapy. Medications include lorezepam for anxiety and sensations of breathlessness.

1. What medications would you suggest for emergency episodes of dyspnea? And what route? What dose?

2. When patient has more difficulty breathing, what would recommendations be?

3. If the patient would like to get a longer acting benzodiazepines what would you suggest?

4. Since the patient is bed bound, what other issues would be important?

5. What would be important issues to educate his family around his death?

6. What could you do for thickened saliva?

7. What medications would be helpful if you want to dry up secretions?

Case Study #14 Answers

1. **Answer**: MSO4 elixir po/sl/sq 5-10 mg q 15 minutes as needed

2. **Answer**: Administer opioids as per order. If sedated use Ritalin to help decrease sedation. Increase bowel regimen.

3. **Answer**: Diazepam 5-10 mg q 4-6 hours

4. **Answer**: Bowel Regimen
   Skin Care
   Sleep Schedule due to inactivity

5. **Answer**: Anticipatory fear for a respiratory death including fear, anxiety, escalating respiratory distress—all symptoms will be managed. Advanced Care Planning around comfort care should be discussed including future infection and other common symptoms and relevant concerns.

6. **Answer**: Guaifenisen 200 mg q 4 hours

7. **Answer**: Any of the following medications would be helpful:
   scopolomine
   Levsin®
   atropine
   Benadryl®

Case Study #15

Ms. A is a 43-year-old with end stage HIV. She has had HIV for 6-7 years. Illnesses have included bouts of PCP, cryptococcal meningitis, cervical cancer, MAI complex. More recently, she has had seizures. Currently, her CD4 count is 16 and viral load is 700. She is no longer taking antiretrovirals, however remains on antiboiotics for C. diff and fungemia. She also has a history of drug abuse and pain management has been an issue.

1. What are some issues to be addressed in terms of long term care?

2. In assessing pain, what would be important elements to consider?

3. How would pain be addressed in response to her history of addiction?

4. What is difference between addiction and tolerance?

Case Study #15 Answers

1. **Answer**:

   a. Advanced Care Planning including DNR/DNI

   b. Where does she want to die?

   c. Who is the support system to address these issues?

2. **Answer**: The typical assessment, which would include, location, duration, intensity, factors which increase or decrease pain, other medications currently prescribed.

3. **Answer**: Separate pain from any methadone maintenance program. May need to contract for medications.

4. **Answer**: Addiction is a primary, chronic, neurobiologic disease, with genetic, psychosocial, and environmental factors influencing its development and manifestations. It is characterized by behaviors that include one or more of the following: impaired control over drug use, compulsive use continued despite harm, and craving (defined by American Pain Foundation Spring 2001 newsletter). Tolerance is a state of adaptation in which exposure to a drug induces changes that result in a diminution of one or more of the drug's effects over time (defined by American Pain Foundation Spring 2001 newsletter).

Case Study #16

Mr. L is a 78-year-old male admitted for head trauma and internal bleeding secondary to a motor vehicle accident. Prior to his accident, Mr. L had some dementia. His wife, his primary caregiver, was driving the car and was killed in the accident. Mr. L's only child, a son, is now the only family member. The son had never been involved in Mr. L's care prior to the accident. Neurologists have told Mr.L's son that the prognosis is very poor. Mr. L will not regain his former function and will be bedbound. Mr. L appears restless and anxious.

1. How should we assess Mr. L's pain?

2. What pain medications should be considered for Mr. L?

3. How should the nurse assess dyspnea?

4. What teaching is important for the son?

5. What care is important at this time?

6. What education will the son need once the ventilator is no longer needed?

Case Study #16 Answers

1. **Answer:** To assess pain, the nurse will have to evaluate vital signs and non-verbal cues. Tachypnea, tachycardia and increases in blood pressure can all signal pain. Staff should also observe non-verbal cues, such as grimacing, body movement, and anxiety.

2. **Answer:** The patient could benefit from morphine, starting with a low dose. The patient is elderly so we need to start low—3 mg IV and titrate up as needed. In addition,Valium® 2-10 mg IV every 4-6 hours will alleviate anxiety. Valium® is a better choice for the elderly since it is longer acting and better tolerated and IV dosing is preferred due to dementia. The morphine would be helpful in alleviating respiratory distress. If upper airway secretions are problematic, scopolamine patches, glycoprrolate nebs or Levsin® tablets may be indicated.

3. **Answer:** One would need to assess respiratory rate and quality, such as snoring, rattling or gasping respirations. Looking at the use of neck muscles and intercostal muscles can help assess the energy needed for each breath. In addition, monitoring oxygen saturation levels and the patient's skin color would be part of the assessment. However, oxygen saturation monitoring is often unnecessary. If the family is having a hard time understanding shortness of breath, have the family member sit at the patient's bedside for 10-15 minutes and have them breath at the same rate as the patient. Often, this helps them feel the fatigue of dyspnea and the secondary lightheadedness.

4. **Answer:** The son needs someone to spend time describing the extent of the injuries, what those injuries might mean in forecasting the patient's best possible outcome, and what will be done to assure the patient's comfort. The team should also assist the son in coping with the situation by assessing his level of understanding, his concerns, his specific needs. In addition, the son needs to understand the dying trajectory.

5. **Answer:** The patient will likely be anxious, so he needs to be spoken to as though he can hear and understand everything. Reassurance is critical as is medication for anxiety if indicated. Keeping the patient relaxed, calm and reassured should be specific goals of the team. Use of benzodiazepines may be needed. In addition, much education is needed. The son needs to be educated about the possible course of the g-tube, in that it may work at first and then there may be residuals and diarrhea requiring that feedings be stopped. In addition, there needs to be constant dialogue about the goal of the ventilator in terms of overall quality of life issues.

6. **Answer:** The son needs to be apprised of all possible scenarios, assured that the patient and family will not be abandoned, that the patient's comfort and dignity will be assured. Specific needs include arrangements for caretakers, tube feedings, tracheostomy suctioning, cleaning and tape changes. Assessment of psychosocial and spiritual needs of the patient and son are very important at this time. In addition, the plan of care for withdrawal of the ventilator needs to be explained. This includes an agreed upon time to carry out the task, who will be there from the health care team, meds to be used, what may happen after the ventilator is withdrawn, realistic expectations particularly that the patient may not die right away or that respiratory distress will be avoided and narcotics used, and what the patient may look like. The son should be offered support of family and clergy at the time of withdrawal.

Case Study #17

Ms. N is a 43-year-old woman with end stage renal failure and peripheral vascular disease. She was admitted for surgery of a non-healing ulcer of her left foot. Post-operatively she developed an infection necessitating a left below knee amputation (BKA). Then complications arose with her right leg and she underwent a right BKA. Soon thereafter, she developed gangrene. Ms. N is now considering whether to undergo more surgery or discontinue all aggressive measures including her dialysis.

1. What pain control should be initiated for painful dressing changes?

2. What dosing adjustments must be considered with her renal failure?

3. If she foregoes dialysis, what would her course be?

4. What adjustments would be necessary for her pain control?

5. What family education regarding her death is necessary?

Case Study #17 Answers

1. **Answer**: The patient should receive intravenous pain medication (morphine or Dilaudid®) 15-30 minutes prior to dressing changes.

2. **Answer:** Dosing should take into account altered metabolism and excretion due to renal failure, so doses may be lower than usual to start, with slower titration and longer intervals. Assess pain levels frequently to determine effectiveness.

3. **Answer**: Usually death occurs within 7-10 days. Patient may be responsive the first 3-4 days and then go into a coma. It depends somewhat on her current BUN, creatinine and potassium levels but with advanced renal failure coupled with gangrene, her decline will no doubt be rapid and progressive. Uremia will occur. Metabolic acidosis will result in confusion, stupor, possible seizures and coma.

4. **Answer:** Mrs. N will need good pain control due to the gangrene and adjuvants may be indicated to manage itching and confusion. However, much less medication is needed since it will not leave the body once dialysis is stopped. Careful dosing is important due to her altered metabolism.

5. **Answer:** Describe the renal death as above. The family needs an estimated time frame so that they can prepare emotionally, spiritually, and financially. They need to be assured that symptoms such as pain, fever, agitation/confusion will be adequately managed, and that death will likely be peaceful, probably ending in coma. Funeral planning support should be offered through members of the interdisciplinary team.

Case Study #18

Mr. L is a 55-year-old male with end-stage cardiomyopathy. His ejection fraction is 10%. He has undergone all possible surgical interventions without improvement. He is currently on a dobutamine drip that is maintaining his blood pressure. He would like to go home to die.

1. What would the discharge plan be?

2. What would you give for pain control?

3. What other medications would be important?

4. What patient/family education is important?

Case Study #18 Answers

1. **Answer**: The patient and family should be given the option of continuing the dobutamine at least long enough to get him home and settled in. He will need someone with him at all times, so that his exertion is minimal. Oxygen, diuretics, antianxiety and pain medicines are all indicated. Once at home the dobutamine can be discontinued and the narcotics initiated.

2. **Answer:** Morphine, as it will also ease dyspnea and air hunger.

3. **Answer:** Primarily benzodiazepines as in the emergency room a patient is treated with narcotics and benzodiazepines so this should be simulated at home. Diuretics, Digoxin® (if patient opts to continue it), anti-anxiety medications such as Ativan® and perhaps a sleeping medication.

4. **Answer:** Family needs to know possible scenarios with this patient, especially the most likely one of pulmonary edema/respiratory distress and/or pneumonia. Discussion should take place about which medications will be used. For some families, oral antibiotics are seen as comfort medications. Otherwise, they need assurance that medicines such as morphine or hydromorphone and Valium® or Ativan® should be given every 15 minutes until comfort is attained. The goal is to assure the patient will not experience any distress and that death could be peaceful and gradual, or could come as the result of a sentinal event (PE, MI, etc).

Case Study #19

Ms. S is a 21-year-old young woman status post multiple liver transplants. Her liver failure began when she was 13. She has undergone two liver transplants. The first one failed three years after the transplant. She is on numerous immunosuppressive medications and states her quality of life is poor and she doesn't want to live like this anymore. She has decided to stop all of her medications.

1. What assessment is necessary of Ms. S and her family?

2. What medications are appropriate for treatment of Ms. S?

3. What information should be given to the family about what Ms. S may experience in her dying process. What preparation hints would you give?

Case Study #19 Answers

1. **Answer**: It is necessary to assess for depression and decision-making capacity. If it is determined she is not depressed and can make decisions, then her choices to discontinue medications should be honored. If that is not the case, one would want to know how Ms S's family feels about her decision. Then it would be important to determine her health care proxy or advanced directive.

2. **Answer:** Ms. S will need medication for pain such as morphine, hydromorphone or oxycodone, for urticaria such as antihistamines, hydrocortisone lotion, or other medications, for fever such as indomethacin suppositories or other liquid NSAIDS, for dyspnea such as pain meds, agitation and for hallucinations from encephalopathy such as Haldol® or Thorazine.

3. **Answer:** The family should be told, gently, that death could follow a lapse into a coma and be peaceful or could occur suddenly as the result of internal bleeding. They should also be told that confusion/agitation and pain are possibilities when dealing with hepatic failure. The family should be guided to have dark towels available in the event of a massive GI bleed. They should be given instructions on how to administer prefilled syringes of morphine and Valium® in the event of a sudden bleed to assure comfort and explain these will not prolong her life but make sure she has no distress.

Case Study #20

E.L. is an 11-year-old Cambodian boy who experienced an anoxic brain injury at the age of 6. He was involved in an accident where he fell under ice for 45 minutes resulting in respiratory arrest. He was found unresponsive. He continued to be unresponsive following pulmonary resuscitation and has lived in a rehabilitation setting in a permanent vegetative state. He has been developing recurrent pneumonias necessitating hospitalizations and aggressive respiratory therapy. Recently, the family has decided his quality of life is poor and they want no further antibiotic therapy.

1. What assessment of the patient and family is indicated?

2. What assessment of the staff is necessary?

3. What signs and symptoms would be attended to in making this boy more comfortable?

4. What medications are necessary to treat these symptoms?

5. What family/staff education is important in this scenario?

Case Study #20 Answers

1. **Answer:** One needs to find an interpreter to convene a family meeting. During this time, one needs to first explore the cultural implications of the death of a young boy and any religious beliefs that are important to this process. Then one needs to ensure that the family understands the outcome of foregoing antibiotics. They should also be assured any subsequent symptoms that occur will be aggressively managed. Finally, if appropriate, the family may want to understand the dying process. The team should explore the spiritual/religious support needed in this case.

2. **Answer:** The staff has become extended family. They need to be given ample opportunity to process the parent's decision and the parent's right to choose this option. It would be good to give detailed explanations of the scenarios that are possible for the boy and how symptoms will be managed. It is important for the palliative care team to allow those uncomfortable with this to support their conscientious objection. Finally, it needs to be impressed upon staff that care has not been withdrawn, rather there is more intensive detail to symptoms. Perhaps, to get buy-in, it would be best to use meds currently being used and not withdraw all treatments at once.

3. **Answer:** This child will likely experience fever, sweats, dyspnea and increased upper airway secretions.

4. **Answer:** Treat the fever with Tylenol® or indomethacin suppositories as they are longer acting. Treat dyspnea with narcotics or nebulized medications such as albuterol or steroids if that is what he has been consistently receiving. For congestion, glycoprrolate nebs, scopolamine, or even IV Benadryl® can help. Finally, IV fluids should be discontinued or decreased to a keep vein open level.

5. **Answer:** Family needs to be assured of non-abandonment, adequate symptom management, preservation of dignity. They need to be offered information and allowed to make choices. Again cultural and spiritual assessment is critical to assure respect and support. Staff needs to be supported through the process. Frequent staff assessment and debriefing after the death may be necessary.

Pharmacology

Definitions

Definition of terms according to the American Pain Foundation Spring 2001 newsletter.

Addiction is a primary, chronic, neurobiologic disease, with genetic, psychosocial, and environmental factors influencing its development and manifestations. It is characterized by behaviors that include one or more of the following: impaired control over drug use, compulsive use continued despite harm, and craving (defined by American Pain Foundation Spring 2001 newsletter).

Physical Dependence is a state of adaptation that is manifested by a drug class specific withdrawal syndrome that can be produced by abrupt cessation, rapid dose reduction, decreasing blood level of the drug, and/or administration of an antagonist (defined by American Pain Foundation Spring 2001 newsletter).

Tolerance is a state of adaptation in which exposure to a drug induces changes that result in a diminution of one or more of the drug's effects over time (defined by American Pain Foundation Spring 2001 newsletter).

Pseudoaddiction was recognized recently after clinicians repeatedly observed that many patients who were labeled as "difficult" and "drug seeking" were actually being undertreated for pain. Factors contributing to pseudoaddiction include prescription of opioids at intervals greater than their expected duration of action, or in doses too low or of insufficient potency for the intensity of their pain. In such cases, patients who have suffered prolonged, unrelieved pain may become more aggressive in seeking relief. The clinician must thoroughly assess the adequacy of the treatment before making a judgment (defined by MD Anderson Cancer Center Nursing Reports on Strategies for Pain Management. Rugu, T.F., Canningham, M. L., Thorpe, D. M. (1998) 1, (2)).

Combination Products

Darvocet-N 50®: acetaminophen 325 mg and propoxyphene napsylate 50 mg (include Darvocet N-100®)

Darvon Compound+®: aspirin 325 mg propoxyphene hydrochloride 32 mg and caffeine 32.4 mg

Darvon Compound-65®: aspirin 389 mg propoxyhene hydrochloride 65 mg and caffeine 32.4 mg

Darvon-N Compound®: aspirin 375 mg propoxyphene napsylate 100 mg and caffeine 30 mg

Fioricet with Codeine®: acetaminophen 325 mg butalbital 50 mg caffeine 40 mg and codeine phosphate 30 mg

Lorcet 10/650®: acetaminophen 650 mg and hydrocodone bitartrate 10 mg

Lortab 5/500®: acetaminophen 500 mg and hydrocodone bitartrate 5 mg

Percodan-Demi®: aspirin 325 mg, oxycodone hydrochloride 2.25 mg and oxycodone terephthalate 0.19 mg

Percodan-Demi+®: aspirin 325 mg and oxycodone hydrochloride 2.5 mg

Roxicet 5/325®; acetaminophen 325 mg and oxycodone hydrochloride 5 mg

Roxilox 5/500®; acetaminophen 500 mg and oxycodone hydrochloride 5 mg

Roxicet Oral Solution:[1] acetaminophen 325 mg and oxycodone hydrochloride 5 mg/5 ml

Tylenol With Codeine No.1®: acetaminophen 300 mg and codeine phosphate 7.5 mg

Tylenol With Codeine No.2®: acetaminophen 300 mg and codeine phosphate 15 mg

Tylenol With Codeine No.3®: acetaminophen 300 mg and codeine phosphate 30 mg

Tylenol With Codeine No.4®: acetaminophen 300 mg and codeine phosphate 60 mg

Tylox®: acetaminophen 500 mg and oxycodone hydrochloride 5 mg

---

1 Liquid form contains alcohol

Common Palliative Pharmacologic Brand Names Followed by Generic Names

Ativan® = lorazepam

Demerol® = meperidine

Dilaudid® = hydromorphone HCL

Dolophine HCL® = methadone

Duragesic® = fentanyl citrate

Halcion® = triazolam

Haldol® = haloperidol

Indocin® = indomethacin

MS Contin® = morphine long acting

MSIR® = morphine intermediate release

Narcan® = naloxone

Oxycontin® = oxycodone long acting

Percodan® = oxycodone HCL

Reglan® = metoclopramide

Roxanol® = morphine elixir

Roxicodone® = oxycodone

Talwin® = pentazocine HCL

Tritisate® = choline magnesium trisalicylate

Tylenol® = acetaminophen

Valium® = diazepam

Vicodan® = hydrocodone bitartrate

Xanax® = alprazolam

Conversions Worksheet

Formula for converting to new drug or new route:

Morphine $\frac{\text{Current 24-hour dose}}{\text{Current equivalent \#}}$ x new equivalent # = new 24-hour dose

For calculating breakthrough dose:

⅙ to ¼ 24-hour dose, avail q 1–2 hour prn

Problem 1. Mr. Hahn is being switched by his doctor from po morphine to po Dilaudid®. The patient is on MS Contin® 100 mg q 8 hours, plus 10 mg MSIR® for prn (used 6 times in 24 hours). What will the patient's q 4 hourly dose of Dilaudid® be?

Problem 2. Mrs. Finley has been on IV morphine, 4 mg/hour. She is now able to take oral meds and will be switched to oral morphine. What will her q 4 hourly dose be?

Problem 3. Mr. Malia is on PO Demerol® 75 mg q 3 hours. He is having increased pain and it is anticipated he will not be able to tolerate side effects of increased Demerol®. If he is switched to MS Contin®, what would his 12-hourly dose be?

Problem 4. Mrs. Swift has had her pain well-controlled on oral Methadone® 20 mg q 6 hours, but her increasing obtundance is thought to be a SE of Methadone rather than from her disease process. You want to suggest a trial of oral Oxycontin® to the doctor, what would be the equivalent q 12 hour dose.

Problem 5. Mrs. Donahue has been receiving Dilaudid® 15 mg PO q 4 hours. Dr. Brown wants her switched to IV morphine because of her difficulty swallowing.

Problem 6. Calculate the breakthrough dose of MSIR® for a patient who is on MS Contin® 120 mg q 12 hours.

Conversions Worksheet Answers

Answer 1.

360	÷	30	=	12	×	7.5	=	90
Current 24-hour dose	÷	Current drug equivalent	=	equianalgesic dose units	×	New drug/route equianalgesic #	=	new 24-hour dose

90 ÷ 6 = 15 mg q 4 hours

Answer 2. 96 ÷ 10 = 9.6 x 30 = 288 — 288 ÷ 6 = 48 mg q 4 hours

Answer 3. 600 ÷ 300 = 2 x 30 = 60 — 60 ÷ 2 = 30 mg q 12 hours

Answer 4. 80 ÷ 20 = 4 x 15 = 60 — 60 ÷ 2 = 30 mg q 12 hours

Answer 5. 90 ÷ 7.5 = 12 x 10 = 120 — 120 ÷ 24 = 5 mg/hours

Answer 6. 240 mg/24 hour

⅙ = 40 mg
¼ = 60 mg

Medication Problem-Solving Questions and Answers

1. Combination analgesics that contain acetaminophen are not recommended for patients with hepatic insufficiency. What combination product would be contraindicated?

   A. Percodan®

   B. Meperidine

   C. Vicodin®

   D. Oxycodone

2. The Cancer Pain Management Guidelines written through the Agency for Health Care Policy and Research (AHCPR) recommends that analgesics be given ________ as the most preferred route.

   A. Parenterally

   B. Rectally

   C. Transdermally

   D. Orally

3. How much oxycodone per day is the patient receiving when taking two Tylox® q 4 hour?

4. How much acetaminophen per day is the patient receiving when taking two Tylox® q 4 hour?

5. What is the maximum recommended number of milligrams of acetaminophen permitted per day?

6. If 20 mg of oxycodone is equivalent to 30 mg morphine then how much morphine is equivalent to 60 mg of oxycodone?

7. Addiction is best described as:

   A. A significant risk for anyone taking opioids for pain

   B. A psychologic problem when drug-seeking and drug-taking behavior become the paramount purposes in life despite significant risk of harm

   C. A phenomenon whereby higher doses of a drug are required over time to maintain the same therapeutic effect

   D. Primarily a physiologic problem in which the patient becomes dependent on the drug.

8. The only NSAID available for parenteral administration is:

   A. Naproxen®

   B. Sulindac®

   C. Ibuprofen®

   D. Ketorolac®

1. Answer is C:

   A. Incorrect—Contains 325 mg aspirin; no acetaminophen.

   B. Incorrect—Contains no acetaminophen.

   C. **Correct**—Contains 500 mg acetaminophen so would be contraindicated in patients with hepatic insufficiency.

   D. Incorrect—Contains no acetaminophen.

2. Answer is D

   A. Incorrect—Injectables are not preferred and should be avoided due to discomfort, inconvenience and unreliability of absorption.

   B. Incorrect—The rectal route should be avoided unless absolutely necessary such as with nausea/vomiting, bowel obstruction or when the patient is fasting for surgery.

   C. Incorrect—Often utilized when the gut is malfunctioning but is not the preferred route due to expense.

   D. **Correct**—"If the gut works, use it," the mantra of pain management, because it is the most convenient and the most cost effective.

3. Answer: One Tylox® equals 5 mg oxycodone and 500 mg acetaminophen
   $2 \times 5\text{mg} = 10\text{ mg} \times 6 = 60$ mg of oxycodone/day.

4. Answer: One Tylox® equals 5 mg oxycodone and 500 mg acetaminophen
   $2 \times 500 = 1{,}000 \times 6 = 6{,}000$ mg of acetaminophen/day.

5. Answer: 4 GM or 4000 mg.

6. Answer: 20 mg oxycodone = 30 mg morphine so 60 mg oxycodone = 90 mg morphine

7. Answer is B

   A. Incorrect—When opioids are taken to relieve physiologic pain, the risk of addiction is minimal.

   B. **Correct**—This is in fact the definition of addiction.

   C. Incorrect—This is the definition for tolerance.

   D. Incorrect—This is the definition for dependence.

8. Answer is D

   A. Incorrect—Not available for parenteral use.

   B. Incorrect—Not available for parenteral use.

   C. Incorrect—Not available for parenteral use.

   D. **Correct**—This is the only NSAID with a parenteral formulation available.

9. The oral equianalgesic dose for 4 mg of hydromorphone (Dilandid®) IV is approximately.

A. 2 mg PO.

B. 4 mg PO.

C. 10 mg PO.

D. 20 mg PO.

10. Convert Dilaudid® 7.5 mg q 3 hour PO to MS Contin®.

A. 240 mg PO bid q 12 hour.

B. 60 mg PO bid q 12 hour.

C. 120 mg PO bid q 12 hour.

D. 900 mg PO bid q 12 hour.

11. Convert morphine 10 mg SQ q 4 hour to the equianalgesic daily dose of Oxycontin® PO (morphine 10 mg equals Oxycontin® 20 mg).

A. 60 mg q 12 hour.

B. 40 mg q 12 hour.

C. 20 mg q 12 hour.

D. 10 mg q 12 hour.

12. The ratio of oxycodone, immediate release, to morphine as recommended by AHCPR guidelines is:

A. 1:1

B. 3:1

C. 1.5:7.5

D. 1:3

9. Answer is D

A. Incorrect—See calculations under answer D.

B. Incorrect—See calculations under answer D.

C. Incorrect—See calculations under answer D.

D. **Correct**
The problem is solved as follows:
Hydromorphone 4 mg IV to be converted to what dose of hydromorphone PO.
We know that Hydromorphone 1.5 mg IV equals hydromorphone 7.5 mg PO therefore the equation is: 4mg: × = 1.5 mg: 7.5 mg (multiply the inner two figures against the outer two figures)
1.5 mg × = 30 mg
= 20 mg hydromorphone PO.

10. Answer is C

A. Incorrect—See calculations under C.

B. Incorrect—See calculations under C.

C. **Correct**
Dilaudid ® 7.5 mg PO = 30 mg PO morphine
7.5 mg × 8 doses (in 24^0) = 60 mg
$\frac{7.5}{30} = 60$ × 7.5 × =1800
240 mg MS Contin® in 24^0 (120 mg PO q12h)

D. Incorrect—See calculations under C.

11. Answer is A

A. **Correct**
Morphine 10 mg SQ q 4 hour is equal to what dose of Oxycontin® 12 hour PO
Morphine 10 mg IV equals 20 mg of Oxycontin® q 12 hour PO. The patient is taking the SQ q 4 hour therefore receives a total of 60 mg of morphine in a 24-hour period.
Therefore the equation is as follows: 60 mg : × = 10 mg : 20 mg
10 × = 1200 mg
× = 120 mg of Oxycontin® in a 24 hour period so the answer would be 60 mg q 12 hours.

B. Incorrect—See calculations under A.

C. Incorrect—See calculations under A.

D. Incorrect—See calculations under A.

12. Answer is A

A. **Correct**—This is the correct ratio for oxycodone and morphine.

B. Incorrect—This is the ratio for oral to parenteral routes.

C. Incorrect—This is the ratio for parenteral to oral equianalgesic conversion for dilaudid.

D. Incorrect—This ratio would be much too high. The correct ratio is 1:1.

13. The most effective combination of drugs to relieve pain due to metastatic bone disease is

A. Hydromorphone® and Diazepam®.

B. Acetaminophen and lorazepam.

C. Morphine and acetaminophen.

D. Ibuprofen and morphine.

14. What is the starting dose of morphine in an opioid-naive patient experiencing dyspnea?

A. 2.5 to 5 mg of oral morphine every 4 hours.

B. 60 mg of MS Contin® every 12 hours

C. 10 mg of SQ morphine every hour.

D. Morphine is not safe to use for dyspnea.

15. First line therapy for pneumocystis carinii pneumonia is:

A. Pentamidine (Nebapent®).

B. Trimethoprim/sulfamethoxazole (Bactrim®).

C. Dapsone (Avlosulfon®).

D. Amphotericin B (Fungizone®).

16. Kayexalate may be used to treat:

A. Hyperkalemia

B. Hypernatremia

C. Hyperphosphotemia

D. Hypercalcemia

13. Answer is D

A. Incorrect—Dilaudid® and Valium® are not a combination for metastatic bone pain.

B. Incorrect—Tylenol® and Ativan® would provide minimum relief for metastatic bone pain.

C. Incorrect—While morphine is the drug of choice, Tylenol® is not the best drug to be used in metastatic bone pain.

D. **Correct**—Morphine with ibuprofen is an NSAID and the drug of choice with Morphine. Ibuprofen is very effective as an adjuvant analgesic agent in combination with morphine for metastatic bone pain (Morphine is limited in it's ability to manage bone pain).

14. Answer is A

A. **Correct**—The opioid naive patient should be started on very low doses of oral morphine to assess the effectiveness without causing side effects of overdosing.

B. Incorrect—Long acting morphine is not the drug of choice for dyspnea.

C. Incorrect—Subcutaneous morphine is not necessary—it is painful, invasive, inconvenient and has a variable absorption rate.

D. Incorrect—Morphine is very safe for dyspnea and in fact is the drug of choice.

15. Answer is B

A. Incorrect—Pentamidine would be second line therapy if first line therapy failed.

B. **Correct**—Trimethoprim/sulfamethoxazole is Bactrim® and is the first line therapy for *pneumocystis carinii* pneumonia.

C. Incorrect—Dapsone is an antibacterial sulfone treatment for leprosy.

D. Incorrect—Amphotericin B is an antifungel agent given IV.

16. Answer is A

A. **Correct—**Kayexalate® is used to treat hyperkalemia since it is a potassium removing resin that exchanges sodium ions for potassium ions in the intestine.

B. Incorrect—Hypernatremia is high sodium and would not benefit from Kayexalate®.

C. Incorrect—Hyperphosphotemia is high phosphorus levels in the serum. Phosphorus compounds are the principle sources of energy in muscle contraction and are essential in the conversion of glycogen to glucose. Hyperphosphotemia would not benefit from Kayexalate®.

D. Incorrect—Hypercalcemia is high serum levels of calcium and would not benefit from Kayexalate®.

17. Headaches caused by increased intracranial pressure would be best treated by:

A. Belladonna

B. Dexamethasone

C. Ibuprofen

D. Nortriptyline

18. Mrs. Brown is currently receiving Oxycontin® 60 mg every 12 hours for metastatic breast carcinoma with mets to pelvis, spine and left femur. She has taken 4 doses of oxycodone 20 mg over the past 24 hours for breakthrough pain. What is the new dose of Oxycontin® that should be initiated to relieve Mrs. Brown's pain?

Long Acting 25-50%

A. 65 mg

B. 70 mg

C. 75 mg

D. 100 mg

19. Mr. Smith has multiple sites of bone metastases from his primary prostate carcinoma. He reports that despite taking Oxycontin 30 mg every 12 hours, his pain level remains at "8" when ambulating. You notice he does not have any breakthrough pain prescriptions. What dose of Oxy IR® would you expect his physician to order? Oxycontin 30 mg equals what dose of Oxy IR® ?

1/6-1/4 of long acting

A. 5 mg

B. 10 mg

C. 15 mg

D. 20 mg

20. Maximum daily dose of Megace® is

A. 200 mg

B. 400 mg

C. 600 mg

D. 800 mg

400mg BID

17. Answer is B

A. Incorrect—Belladonna is an antispasmotic and would be inappropriate in this case.

B. **Correct**—Dexamethasone is a steroidal agent and is best to treat increased intracranial pressure caused by swelling.

C. Incorrect—Ibuprofen is an NSAID (nonsteroidal anti-inflammatory drug) that would not relieve increased intracranial pressure.

D. Incorrect—Nortriptyline (Pamelor®) is an antidepressant that would not relief the headache caused by increased intracranial pressure.

18. Answer is D

A. Incorrect—An additional 10 mg/24 hours would be insufficient.

B. Incorrect—An additional 20 mg/24 hours still would be insufficient.

C. Incorrect—While 25 % of the daily dose may be the first level of titration, in this situation Mrs. Brown required more breakthrough indicating an increase of 50% for proper titration is needed.

D. **Correct**—Titrate by increasing the dose 25–50%; do not increase frequency
Titration is done by percentages
never less than 25% (mild pain)
mild—moderate Pain (1-6/10), 25-50%
severe pain (7—10/10), 50-100%.

19. Answer is B

A. Incorrect—Insufficient dose for breakthrough.

B. **Correct**—Breakthrough dose should be 1/6 of 24-hour Oxycontin® dose.

C. Incorrect—This dose would be more than is indicated.

D. Incorrect—This dose would be more than is indicated.

20. Answer is D

A. Incorrect—Megace® is normally given in doses of 400 mg bid.

B. Incorrect—This is a one time dose of Megace®—it is normally given 400 mg twice a day.

C. Incorrect—Megace® can be given to a level of 800 mg a day.

D. **Correct**—The maximum daily dose of Megace® is 800 mg. It is normally prescribed as Megace® 400 mg bid.

21. Medications that can color urine, feces, sputum, sweat, and tears a red-orange color and stain soft contact lenses are:

A. Dapson (Aviosulfon®) and pentamidine (Nebupent®)

B. Isoniazid (INH®) and ethambutol (Myambutol®)

C. Rifabutin (Mycobutin®) and rifampin (Rifadin®)

D. Azithouromycin (Zithromax®) and clarithromycin (Biaxin®)

22. Which of the following pain medications must not be crushed?

A. Morphine sulfate SR

B. Acetaminophen (Tylenol®) with codeine

C. Percocet®/Percodan®

D. Hydromorphone (Dilaudid®)

23. A "ceiling dose" of a medication is:

A. The maximum dose giving therapeutic results without undesirable side effects

B. The maximum safe dose to prevent respiratory depression

C. The highest dose the pharmacy will dispense

D. The highest dose in which the drug is manufactured

24. Patients taking narcotics on a regular schedule must:

A. Wake themselves at night to prevent respiratory depression

B. Adjust the amount of medication they use depending on the time of day

C. Plan to wean themselves off narcotics as soon as possible

D. Be placed on a daily bowel regimen to prevent constipation

21. Answer is C

A. Incorrect—Dapsone is used to treat Leprosy and pentamidine is used in the treatment of pneumocystis carinii pneumonia. Neither of these agents cause discolorations of bodily secretions.

B. Incorrect—Although both of these agents treat pulmonary tuberculosis, neither cause discolorations of bodily secretions.

C. **Correct**—The antitubercular agents, Mycobutin® and Rifadin® or their metabolites, can permanently stain soft contact lenses and will discolor urine, feces, sputum, sweat and tears.

D. Incorrect—Both agents are macrolide anti-infectives but neither cause discoloration of bodily secretions.

22. Answer is A

A. **Correct**—SR means sustained release. Sustained release products lose their effect if crushed.

B. Incorrect—Tylenol® with codeine can be crushed without loss of effect.

C. Incorrect—Percocet® or Percodan® could be crushed without losing any effect.

D. Incorrect—Hydromorphone can be crushed without causing loss of effect.

23. Answer is A

A. **Correct**—Ceiling dose refers to the maximum dose giving therapeutic results without undesirable side effects.

B. Incorrect—Respiratory depression would be one but not the only undesirable side effects of a medication.

C. Incorrect—The pharmacy will dispense whatever dose the physician orders within the norm of that medication. If any discrepancies occur, the pharmacist is required to contact the physician for clarification.

D. Incorrect—The ceiling dose is not the highest dose manufactured.

24. Answer is D

A. Incorrect—Patients may need to wake themselves at night to take their medication to assure around the clock administration, however they do not need to wake themselves to prevent respiratory depression. Respiratory depression is caused by too much medication. The resulting somnolence would prevent waking oneself.

B. Incorrect—Excessive amounts of medication is the cause of respiratory depression not the time of the day.

C. Incorrect—Decreasing the amount of medication should be due to relief of discomfort from some other intervention. The patient taking narcotics should consider decreasing the dose as the pain levels decrease and no longer require the current dose levels.

D. **Correct**—All patients taking narcotics should be placed on a daily bowel regimen because constipation is the one side effect that is experienced by all and should be prevented.

25. Nonsteroidal anti-inflammatory drugs (NSAIDs) may be used alone or with narcotics, specifically for:

A. Neuropathic pain

B. Bone pain

C. Visceral pain

D. Abdominal pain

26. For the patient with persistent pain from metastatic cancer, pain medications should be given:

A. PRN to avoid addiction and tolerance

B. Four times daily

C. Via a patch or intravenously for more severe pain

D. Around the clock on a regular schedule; plus a prn dose for breakthrough pain

27. Why are phenothiazines commonly used as narcotic adjuvants for chronic pain?

A. Antianxiety activity

B. Antiemetic activity

C. Analgesic activity

D. A and B above

28. For patients placed on SR (sustained-release) narcotics for chronic pain relief, which of the following drugs would be an appropriate choice for acute "breakthrough" pain?

A. Pentazocine (Talwin®)

B. Hydromorphone (Dilaudid®)

C. Butorphanol (Stadol®)

D. Nalbuphine (Nubain®)

25. Answer is B

A. Incorrect—Neuropathic pain responds to anticonvulsants such as neurontin but not NSAIDs since it is caused by peripheral or central nervous system nerve injury.

B. **Correct**—Bone pain is secondary to inflammation and therefore very responsive to the nonsteroidal anti-inflammatory drugs.

C. Incorrect—Visceral pain results from direct stimulation to intact afferent nerve endings in the viscera and therefore is most responsive to opioids.

D. Incorrect—Abdominal pain is usually visceral pain reflective of organ stimulation and therefore responds most effectively to opioids.

26. Answer is D

A. Incorrect—Patients experiencing persistent pain should always receive around the clock medications to assure a consistent blood level. PRN medications should be used for breakthrough pain.

B. Incorrect—Administering pain medications four times a day may be insufficient to control pain around the clock especially if the scheduling is during the waking hours only.

C. Incorrect—Patches and intravenous pain medication administration are justified only in specific situations. Around the clock oral opioids is the method of choice.

D. **Correct**—The best method of managing pain control in the patient with persistent pain from metastatic cancer is to administer medications around the clock on a regular schedule and offer a prn dose for breakthrough pain.

27. Answer is D

A. Incorrect—Although phenothiazines offer antianxiety benefits, they also offer antiemetic activity as well.

B. Incorrect—Although phenothiazines offer antiemetic benefits, they also offer antianxiety activity as well.

C. Incorrect—Phenothiazines do not offer analgesic activity.

D. **Correct**—Phenothiazines are used commonly as narcotic adjuvants because they offer antianxiety and antiemetic activity.

28. Answer is B

A. Incorrect—Pentazocine (Talwin®) is an opioid agonist-antagonist and therefore may produce withdrawal symptoms if mixed with opioids, have an analgesic ceiling and may have psychomimetic side effects.

B. **Correct**—Hydromorphone (Dilaudid®) is an opioid and very effective as a breakthrough analgesic with sustained release narcotics.

C. Incorrect—Butorphanol (Stadol®) is an opioid agonist-antagonist and therefore may produce withdrawal symptoms if mixed with opioids. It has an analgesic ceiling and may have psychomimetic side effects.

D. Incorrect—Nalbuphine (Nubain®) is an opioid agonist-antagonist and therefore may produce withdrawal symptoms if mixed with opioids. It has an analgesic ceiling and may have psychomimetic side effects.

29. Mr. S rates his pain as 2 to 4 (on the 0-to 10-point pain scale) but insists on the need for stronger medication (a narcotic) or some new plan to relieve his pain. The basis for your response is:

A. That pain at 2 does not require further intervention

B. That Mr. S is being unrealistic in expecting total relief

C. That Mr. S's lack of willingness to tolerate pain at 2 directs the plan

D. That the risks of narcotic use are not warranted in this situation.

30. Which of the following narcotic analgesics is usually NOT preferred in chronic pain minimally due to the drug's short duration of action and toxic metabolites?

A. Meperidine (Demerol®)

B. Morphine

C. Aspirin

D. Methadone

31. Neuropathic pain, which the patient might describe as burning, tingling or shooting, would best be treated with which type of drug?

A. Opioid

B. Nonsteroidal anti-inflammatory drug (NSAID)

C. Tricyclic antidepressant

D. Skeletal muscle relaxant

32. If the patient has a brain tumor and headache that may be caused from edema around the tumor, a useful medication to add to the current analgesic regime would be:

A. Dexamethasone (Decadron®)

B. Phenobarbital

C. Hydrochlorothiazide (HydroDiuril®)

D. Acetaminophen (Tylenol®)

29. Answer is C

A. Incorrect—If Mr. S is requesting stronger medication, we must respond. Margo McCaffery defines pain as "pain is what the patient says it is."

B. Incorrect—Mr. S must define to us his level of acceptance and our plan of care should reflect achievement of that level of acceptance.

C. **Correct**—Mr. S has indicated he will not accept a level of two to four and we must seek the medication dose and schedule that will achieve satisfaction to Mr. S.

D. Incorrect—Adjustments in the type, dose and scheduling of analgesics inclusive of narcotics is required to achieve the acceptable level of comfort for Mr. S.

30. Answer is A

A. **Correct**—Meperidine (Demerol®) has a short duration of only two to three hours. Repeated doses may also lead to central nervous toxicity due to an accumulation of the metabolites called normeperidine.

B. Incorrect—Morphine is the opioid of choice for best analgesic response.

C. Incorrect—Aspirin is not a narcotic.

D. Incorrect—Methadone® has a long duration of action (6-8 hours).

31. Answer is C

A. Incorrect—Neuropathic pain does not respond well to opioids.

B. Incorrect—NSAID best relieve bone pain not neuritic-type pain.

C. **Correct**—Tricyclic antidepressants such as amitriptyline, doxepin, imipramine, and nortriptyline are the agents of choice in neuritic-type pain.

D. Incorrect—Skeletal muscle relaxants would best relieve muscle spasms not nerve pain.

32. Answer is A

A. **Correct**—Cerebral edema is very responsive to corticosteroids. Decadron produces beneficial effects within an hour of the dose administration.

B. Incorrect—Phenobarbital is a barbiturate that depresses monosynaptic and polysynaptic transmission in the CNS and increases the threshold for seizure activity in the motor cortex.

C. Incorrect—Hydrochlorothiazide (HydroDiuril®) is a thiazide diuretic that increases sodium and water excretion by inhibiting sodium and chloride reabsorption in the nephron's distal segment.

D. Incorrect—Acetaminophen (Tylenol®) is thought to produce analgesia by inhibiting prostaglandin synthesis in the CNS but would have little to no benefit with cerebral edema.

33. If a patient is on morphine sulfate 20 mg four times per day and states that it gives good pain relief but that the relief only lasts for 3 hours and the pain always returns before time for the next dose, the following should be considered:

A. Change the morphine sulfate dose to every 3 hours

B. Increase the dose of morphine sulfate

C. Change to a different analgesic

D. Add diazepam (Valium®) to relax the patient

34. The fentanyl transdermal (Duragesic®) patch is subcutaneously absorbed analgesia and:

A. Is routinely changed every 72 hours

B. Absorbs better on skin over some adipose or muscle tissue

C. Can be changed every 48 hours if the patient consistently has increased pain on the third day

D. All of the above

35. Mr. J has severe chemotherapy induced stomatitis and esophagitis. Appropriate intervention would include:

A. Clear liquid diet

B. Lemon-glycerin swab prn

C. Nonsteroidal anti-inflammatory drugs (NSAIDs)

D. Viscous lidocaine (Xylocaine®) 2%-swab mouth every 2 to 3 hours prn

36. The drug of choice in addition to anticonvulsants for treating an active seizure in a terminally ill patient is:

A. Diazepam (Valium®)

B. Amitriptyline (Elavil®)

C. Prochlorperazine (Compazine®)

D. Prednisone

33. Answer is A

A. **Correct**—When the patient defines the period of time that the medication is effective, the scheduling of that medication should correspond if allowable.

B. Incorrect—The dose should not be increased until the maximum allowable scheduling has failed.

C. Incorrect—A different analgesic is not indicated in this situation since the Morphine is effective.

D. Incorrect—Adding diazepam (Valium®) is not advisable especially in the elderly. Diazepam should not be used in the elderly and debilitated patients because they may be more susceptible to the adverse CNS effects of the drug and because it interacts with other common drug therapies such as cimetidine and digoxin.

34. Answer is D

A. Incorrect—Normally the Duragesic patch should be changed every 72 hours. Other answers are also correct.

B. Incorrect—Duragesic® does absorb better on skin over some adipose or muscle tissue. Other answers are correct also.

C. Incorrect—The Duragesic® patch can be changed every 48 hours if the patient consistently has pain on the third day. The other answers are also correct.

D. **Correct**—The best answer for this question is all of the above.

35. Answer is D

A. Incorrect—Clear liquid diet would not offer relief of the discomfort Mr. J is having.

B. Incorrect—Lemon-glycerin swabs would cause additional discomfort.

C. Incorrect—NSAIDs are effective with decreasing bone pain but would offer little relief for mucous membrane discomfort.

D. **Correct**—Xylocaine® viscous 2% would provide a great deal of relief. Offering this intervention every 2 to 3 hours would be helpful until the neutrophils and epithelial cells rebound sufficiently and the stomatitis and esophagitis would disappear.

36. Answer is A

A. **Correct**—Valium®® is a prn order made available to treat a seizure activity which occurs with a terminally ill patient who is currently being treated with anticonvulsants.

B. Incorrect—Elavil® is an antidepressant and would offer no benefit to seizure activity in the terminally ill.

C. Incorrect—Compazine® is an antiemetic and would offer no benefit and is contraindicated with CNS depression.

D. Incorrect—Prednisone, as a corticosteroid, would offer no benefit in this situation.

37. Dyspnea, in a patient with lung cancer, is best treated with:

A. Oxygen by nasal cannula

B. Low-dose morphine

C. Theophylline®

D. Aminophylline®

38. Intractable hiccups may be best treated with:

A. Ondansetron (Zofran®)

B. Phenytoin (Dilantin®)

C. Megesterol (Megace®)

D. Chlorpromazine (Thorazine®)

39. The most appropriate drug for agitation associated with physical harm by the patient to self or others, and/or psychotic tendencies is:

A. Prochlorperazine (Compazine®)

B. Morphine sulfate

C. Haloperidol (Haldol®)

D. Dexamethasone (Decadron®)

40. All EXCEPT one of the following drugs are indicated to control nausea:

A. Prochlorperazine (Compazine®)

B. Dextroamphetamine (Dexedrine®) stimulant

C. Haloperidol (Haldol®)

D. Metoclopramide (Reglan®)

37. Answer is B

A. Incorrect—Oxygen may offer psychological support but would not help physiologically.

B. **Correct**—Low-dose morphine (5 mg SC or PO q 3 hours prn) reduces inappropriate tachypnea and overventilation of the large airways, making breathing more efficient and without carbon dioxide retention. For the opioid-naïve patient, begin with 2.5-5 mg dose. Subcutaneous absorption with only 10-13%.

C. Incorrect—Theophylline®, as a bronchodilator, would only be helpful if the patient has a history of COPD in which this agent was beneficial.

D. Incorrect—Aminophylline® is another bronchodilator that would only be helpful if the patient has a history of COPD.

38. Answer is D

A. Incorrect—Ondansetron (Zofran®) is a selective antagonist of a specific type of serotonin receptor located in the CNS and therefore is an antiemetic used to prevent nausea and vomiting associated with emetogenic chemotherapy.

B. Incorrect—Phenytoin (Dilantin®) is an anticonvulsant which offers no benefit for intractable hiccups.

C. Incorrect—Megesterol (Megace®) is a progestin that changes a neoplastic tumor's hormonal environment thereby altering the neoplastic process. This mechanism does stimulate appetite but has no benefit for intractable hiccups.

D. **Correct**—Chlorpromazine (Thorazine®) is one of the drugs of choice for intractable hiccups caused by stress to the diaphragm, which may be chemical, mechanical or neurological. A dose of 25 mg PO or PR TID is recommended.

39. Answer is C

A. Incorrect—Prochlorperazine (Compazine®) is an antiemetic contraindicated with those patients with CNS depression.

B. Incorrect—Morphine Sulfate is an opioid analgesic that offers little benefit for confusion and agitation unless the agitation is due to a pain syndrome.

C. **Correct**—Haloperidol (Haldol®) is an antipsycotic that blocks postsynaptic dopamine receptors in the brain. Recommended dose is 0.5–5 mg PO q 6-24 hours. Elderly patients usually require lower initial doses and a more gradual dosage titration.

D. Incorrect—Dexamethasone (Decadron®) is a corticosteroid which is recommended for treating cerebral edema and the prevention of seizure activity which may occur secondarily.

40. Answer is B

A. Incorrect—Compazine® is an antiemetic but so is Haldol® and Reglan®.

B. **Correct**—Dextroamphetamine (Dexedrine®) is a CNS stimulant.

C. Incorrect—Haldol® has antiemetic activity although it is primarily an antipsycotic agent.

D. Incorrect—Reglan® is an antiemetic.

General References

Ferrell, B.R. & Coyle, N. (2001). *Textbook of palliative nursing*. Oxford: Oxford University Press.

Hospice Nurses Association. (1995). *Standards of hospice nursing practice and professional performance.* Pittsburgh: Author.

Kuebler, K.K., Dahlin, C.M., Ladd, L., Montonye, M., & Zeri, K. (1996). *Hospice and palliative care clinical practice protocol: Dyspnea*. Pittsburgh: Hospice Nurses Association.

Kuebler, K.K., (1997) *Hospice and palliative care are clinical practice protocol: Terminal Restlessness.* Pittsburgh: Hospice and Palliative Nurses Association.

McCorkle, R., Grant, M., Frank-Stromberg, M., & Baird, S.B. (1996). *Cancer nursing: A comprehensive textbook* (2nd ed.) Philadelphia: WB Saunders.

National Hospice Organization. (1996). *Hospice operations manual.* Arlington, VA: Author.

National Hospice Organization. (1996). *Medical guidelines for determining prognosis in selected non-cancer diseases* (2nd ed.). Arlington, VA: Author

Sheehan, D.C., & Forman, W.B. (1996). *Hospice and palliative care: Concepts and practice*. Boston: Jones & Bartlett.

Sheehan, J.E. (1999) *Hospice and palliative care clinical practice protocol: Nausea and vomiting*. Pittsburgh: Hospice and Palliative Nurses Association.

Smith, S. (2001) *Treatment of end stage non-cancer diagnoses*. Pittsburgh: Hospice and Palliative Nurses Association.

Volker, B.G. (1999) *Hospice and palliative nursing practice review* (3rd ed.). Pittsburgh: Hospice and Palliative Nurses Association.

Volker, B.G. & Watson, A. *Core curriculum for the generalist hospice and palliative nurses* (In print). Pittsburgh: Hospice and Palliative Nurses Association.

Varricchio, C., Pierce, M., Walker, C.L., & Ades, T.B. (1997). *A cancer source book for nurses* (7th ed.). Georgia: American Cancer Society.